When Bad Policy Makes Good Politics

BUSINESS/SCIENCE/TECHNOLOGY DIVISION
CHICAGO PUBLIC LIBRARY
400 SOUTH STATE STREET
CHICAGO, IL 60605

Studies in Postwar American Political Development
Steven Teles, Series Editor

Series Board Members:
Jennifer Hochschild
Desmond King
Sanford Levinson
Taeku Lee
Shep Melnick
Paul Pierson
John Skrentny
Adam Sheingate
Reva Siegel
Thomas Sugrue

When Bad Policy Makes Good Politics

Running the Numbers on Health Reform

ROBERT P. SALDIN

OXFORD
UNIVERSITY PRESS

Oxford University Press is a department of the University of Oxford. It furthers
the University's objective of excellence in research, scholarship, and education
by publishing worldwide. Oxford is a registered trade mark of Oxford University
Press in the UK and certain other countries.

Published in the United States of America by Oxford University Press
198 Madison Avenue, New York, NY 10016, United States of America.

© Oxford University Press 2017

All rights reserved. No part of this publication may be reproduced, stored in
a retrieval system, or transmitted, in any form or by any means, without the
prior permission in writing of Oxford University Press, or as expressly permitted
by law, by license, or under terms agreed with the appropriate reproduction
rights organization. Inquiries concerning reproduction outside the scope of the
above should be sent to the Rights Department, Oxford University Press, at the
address above.

You must not circulate this work in any other form
and you must impose this same condition on any acquirer.

CIP data is on file at the Library of Congress
ISBN 978–0–19–025544–2 (pbk.)
ISBN 978–0–19–025543–5 (hbk.)

9 8 7 6 5 4 3 2 1

Paperback Printed by Webcom, Inc., Canada

Hardback Printed by Bridgeport National Bindery, Inc., United States of America

R0451165637

CHICAGO PUBLIC LIBRARY

For Erin

CONTENTS

ACKNOWLEDGMENTS

This book emerged out of my time in the Robert Wood Johnson Foundation's Scholars in Health Policy Research Program. The two years I spent at Harvard University allowed me to learn about American health policy and explore an interest that I otherwise would not have been able to pursue. I'm grateful to the RWJF for that opportunity and the generous financial support. I would also like to thank my fellow scholars from Cohorts 16, 17, and 18, Kathy Swartz, the longtime leader of the Harvard site, and Alan Cohen, the program director.

Dozens of individuals agreed to speak with me, often at great length and on multiple occasions, about the CLASS Act's development. Their insights proved invaluable. Many colleagues offered helpful comments on various drafts of this book, including Andrea Campbell, Dan DiSalvo, David Mayhew, Rob Mickie, Kris Miler, Jim Morone, Harold Pollack, Patty Strach, and two anonymous reviewers arranged by Steve Teles and Dave McBride at Oxford University Press. Many others offered feedback following presentations at various RWJF conferences and seminars, the 2014 Congress and History Conference at the University of Maryland, and a talk at Montana State University. Publication of this book was also supported by a grant from the Baldridge Book Subvention Fund in the College of Humanities and Sciences at the University of Montana.

Finally, I would like to thank my family, and a few members in particular. My parents have provided years of love and support. This project, however, owes a special debt to my mom. It was her passion and dedication as the founder of a nonprofit organization assisting family caregivers that originally inspired my interest in America's system of long-term care. A special thank you also goes to Erin, who has provided continuous love and support, not to mention several rounds of comments on various drafts. And last but certainly not least, Sylvie and Frankie, who arrived on the scene mid-project, have been a new source of love and joy.

Introduction

They gave up: It was a mess. On October 14, 2011, the Obama admin-istration announced that it was abandoning its efforts to implement a relatively unknown but fiscally significant component of the president's historic health reform law. Department of Health and Human Services Secretary Kathleen Sebelius explained: "It was with the hope of giving Americans better choices that Congress included" the program in the Patient Protection and Affordable Care Act. "Since then," she contin-ued, "our department has worked steadily to find a financially sustain-able model for [it]. . . . Recognizing the enormous need in this country for [this type of offering], we cast as wide a net as possible." But the program, Sebelius said, was fundamentally flawed.[1]

Health reform's boosters in the intellectual class likewise conceded that this piece of the new law was indefensible. Ezra Klein of the *Washington Post*, for instance, acknowledged that "[t]he Obama Administration did the right thing here." Likewise, *Mother Jones'* Kevin Drum admitted that "The budget forecasts for [the program] were always dodgy." And Jonathan Cohn of *The New Republic* confessed that those "who criticized [it] as unsustainable were right to raise alarms, while liberals like me were wrong to ignore them."[2] Congress formally repealed the measure in 2013.

The jettisoned program—the Community Living Assistance Services and Supports (or CLASS) Act—was supposed to help address America's looming long-term care crisis by offering a new self-financing public option for long-term care insurance. It had been championed by Senator

Edward Kennedy (D-MA), and it had been devised by a band of advocates for the disabled and the aging who were working with his staff. But the viability of CLASS had always been in doubt. During health reform's legislative drafting process in 2009–2010, CLASS' design problems spurred widespread, bipartisan allegations that the program amounted to what one Democratic senator called a "Ponzi scheme."[3] The central problem, its critics alleged, was that the purportedly self-sustaining CLASS Act was structured in a manner that would lead to a classic "insurance death spiral" of rising costs and declining enrollments. This meant that keeping it afloat would require tens of billions of dollars in bailouts.

Yet in the midst of the health reform debate, CLASS also had staunch defenders. Most prominently, the White House and Senate Majority Leader Harry Reid (D-NV) insisted that it remain in the legislative package. And the highly respected Congressional Budget Office (CBO) reported that CLASS was anything but the fiscal liability its critics alleged. On the contrary, the CBO projected that CLASS would actually *save* $72 billion, a figure accounting for more than half of the total savings credited to the Affordable Care Act.[4] And, as will be seen, CLASS' CBO-certified savings came to play an important role in the passage of the Affordable Care Act.

But less than two years later, Sebelius issued her statement announcing the Obama administration's reversal on CLASS. Pointing to the same fundamental flaws identified by CLASS' critics during the lawmaking process, she said that the administration had "not identified a way to make CLASS work."[5] A congressional staffer closely involved with the health reform process was less circumspect: "It is unfathomable that people could look at it and think it would work. It was never plausible."[6]

If CLASS was indeed as bad as its detractors claimed and many of its supporters eventually conceded, it is hardly surprising that the Obama administration decided to drop it. Rather, the surprise lies in how a program plagued by widely acknowledged design flaws managed to find its way into the Affordable Care Act in the first place. In fact, beyond its design issues, several other factors made CLASS' inclusion in the health reform law puzzling. First, the American political system—characterized by a separation of powers, checks and balances, a bicameral legislative branch, and various procedural mechanisms that allow minorities to thwart legislation—is notorious for making it difficult to enact even the most well-crafted and popular policies. Second, today's policymaking environment is widely criticized for partisan polarization, gridlock, and a general inability to get anything done. Third, prior to and during the legislative process that produced the Affordable Care Act, sentiment was widespread in Washington—particularly among key supporters of health reform—that long-term care in general, and CLASS in particular, should be addressed separately and were not suitable for the Obamacare package. This factor alone, according to seasoned advocate and scholar Judy Feder, rendered CLASS' inclusion in the Affordable Care Act "miraculous."[7]

The CLASS saga is all the more confounding because the American policymaking process has been revolutionized in the last half century in a way that was supposed to prevent fundamentally flawed policies from becoming law. Beginning in 1974, new safeguards were put in place to ensure fiscal accountability and prevent the kind of free-wheeling policymaking environment that had contributed to alarming budget deficits over the preceding decade. Among these "good government" reforms was the creation of the CBO, a new agency tasked with producing credible financial data to better inform the policymaking process. These changes were widely hailed as ushering in a new era of accountability in Washington.

Given all this, how did CLASS—of all things—manage to overcome this formidable array of obstacles and become law? Why was it designed in a blatantly problematic way? And why would the inclusion of a fundamentally flawed program help ensure passage of arguably the most important social policy legislation since the 1960s?

AMERICA'S LONG-TERM CARE CHALLENGE

Whatever may be said about CLASS' design, it was—without a doubt—targeted at a serious problem. Long-term care encompasses those services and supports that twelve million chronically ill or disabled Americans need to complete basic activities of daily living, such as eating, bathing, getting in and out of bed, and getting dressed. Significant variation exists in terms of level of need, types of services and supports provided, and the location in which this form of care is administered. For individuals with relatively modest limitations, in-home visits by an aide for a few hours a week may be sufficient. At the other end of the spectrum are individuals living in nursing homes and requiring around-the-clock assistance. Although people of any age may require long-term care, the likelihood increases greatly with age. Roughly two-thirds of those needing this form of assistance are sixty-five years of age or older.[8]

Long-term care has been recognized as a serious policy challenge in the United States since around the time of Medicare's enactment. In fact, it was one of the types of coverage that was considered but ultimately dropped from the final Medicare legislation that was signed by President Lyndon B. Johnson to create a national health insurance program for senior citizens. In the decades since, and with Americans living longer, the issue has become even more challenging because the need for long-term care is so closely tied to aging. Demographic forecasts indicate a sharp increase in need in the coming decades as baby boomers age. Already one in eight Americans is at least sixty-five years old, and by 2030 it will be almost one in five. By 2050, forecasts suggest that the current population of people requiring long-term care will more than double. On average, Americans who reach the age of sixty-five can now expect to live to be nearly eighty-four years old. And here's perhaps the most ominous estimate: Of those reaching the age of sixty-five, about 70 percent will need some long-term care, with the average individual requiring three years of assistance.[9]

Traditionally, the overwhelming majority of long-term care in the United States has been provided informally by family members, often at great financial, physical, and emotional cost. Yet just as the need for care is rising, shifts in social trends are eroding this foundation. For instance, recent decades have seen women leaving the home en masse to enter the paid labor force, a rise in single-parent families, a decrease in average family size, and more geographically dispersed families. These and other societal shifts have resulted in fewer adults being available to provide informal long-term care. As a result, many families have increasingly had to seek out paid care.[10]

Paying for long-term care, however, is a concern for individuals, families, and society because it is expensive. A total of 80 percent of national long-term care spending is on elderly recipients. A bed in a nursing home averages between $81,030 (for a shared room) and $90,520 (for a private room) annually, while home health aides average $21 an hour. Nationally, about $220 billion is spent on long-term care each year, amounting to approximately 9 percent of total U.S. health expenditures. And that figure does not even count the $450 billion worth of unpaid care informally provided by family members.[11]

Not surprisingly, these costs become prohibitive for many individuals and families sooner or later. When an individual's financial resources are sufficiently depleted, Medicaid—the only public source of long-term care financing—kicks in. However, once one qualifies for Medicaid, the financial burden is then merely shifted from the individual to society. Medicaid is jointly funded by the states and the federal government, and the program covers 61 percent of all long-term care funding nationally (see Figure 1.1). The program's spending on long-term care has risen dramatically in recent decades. In 1997, Medicaid spent $56 billion on long-term care; by 2011 it was spending $127 billion. Now, a full third of Medicaid's budget goes to financing these services and supports.[12] This sharp rise in spending has created significant pressure on the states because Medicaid is consuming an increasingly large portion of their budgets (see Appendix). Recent studies by the National Conference of State Legislatures have routinely demonstrated that Medicaid is the leading concern for state legislative budget experts.[13] And with millions of baby boomers crossing the senior citizen threshold each year, projections of long-term care needs in the coming decades are staggering, threatening to overwhelm governmental resources and capabilities and crowd out other state-level spending priorities, including education at both the K-12 and university levels, public assistance, corrections, parks and recreation, and transportation.[14]

For many individuals requiring long-term care, the nation's reliance on Medicaid is also problematic. Because Medicaid is means-tested, qualifying for coverage requires elders to "spend down" their savings and become impoverished. Typically, individuals cannot have more than $2,000 in

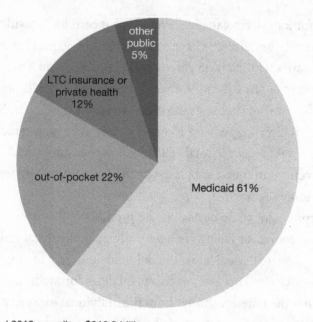

Total 2012 spending: $219.9 billion
* Medicare only pays for limited post-acute care, and is not included here.

Figure 1.1 U.S. Long-Term Care Spending by Payer (2012)

assets, while couples are limited to $3,000 (though primary homes are exempt).[15] Spending down one's financial assets means spending them on their long-term care needs. Giving away money to family members is prohibited, and Medicaid applicants requiring nursing home care are subject to a five year "look back" period to ensure no such transfers of wealth occurred.[16] These eligibility requirements often hit the middle class especially hard. In contrast to poor Americans with few assets to spend down and the wealthy, who can self-finance, those in the vast middle can be financially devastated. For middle-class Americans expecting to pass on modest inheritances to children and grandchildren, long-term care costs can quickly deplete a lifetime of savings. By the time one is eligible for Medicaid, virtually nothing is left.

Private long-term care insurance is available, but the market is dysfunctional. Technical and information problems constrain both insurance providers and potential buyers, yielding expensive policies that only 10 percent of Americans purchase. A typical private long-term care plan has an average monthly premium of about $185 and daily benefits of about $160 for five years.[17] Medicaid's safety-net role as "payer of last resort" decreases demand for private insurance. That is because Medicaid levies "an implicit tax" on private insurance by decreasing the chances of qualifying for Medicaid benefits and extending the time it takes to do so.[18] Recent years have seen private insurance enrollments decline as some companies have quit offering this form of coverage. For the 90 percent of Americans over the age of fifty-five lacking this form of insurance, paying for long-term care often leaves them and their families in economic ruin.

Despite all this, and making the problem all the more acute, Americans are largely ignorant of long-term care. A recent public opinion poll conducted by the Associated Press is only one recent indicator of how ill-prepared the country is for meeting its long-term care challenge. The poll assessed the views of Americans aged forty and older and found low levels of planning for the future or awareness of the costs. Two-thirds of respondents reported little or no planning for their potential needs, and only one-third had saved money. Alarmingly, nearly 40 percent reported not being concerned at all about their future long-term care needs. The poll also indicated problematic assumptions about how long-term care is financed. A total of 42 percent of respondents mistakenly assumed that Medicare will pay nursing home bills while another third erroneously said they expect their health insurance to pick up the tab. Only 17 percent anticipated relying on Medicaid.[19] In sum, the vast majority of Americans have little to no understanding of the financial risks associated with aging.

INCENTIVIZING THE DEVELOPMENT OF BAD POLICY

The advocates who designed CLASS were attempting to address this crisis. Their effort wasn't the first. Prior to CLASS, several plans for creating a national long-term care program had crashed and burned in the 1980s and 1990s. In the years between the last of those failures and the Obama health reform effort, long-term care had been marginalized in Washington policy circles. For those who were aware of the issue, concern remained universal and its importance undisputed. But a viable policy solution was frustratingly elusive.[20] According to the advocates who have worked in the trenches in pursuit of a national program, three stumbling blocks have made it impossible to mobilize public or political support for this worthy cause. First, Americans ignore the situation; people are simply unwilling to face the uncomfortable reality that their golden years will likely entail more than golf courses and cruise ships. Second, as the polling data cited above indicates, a pervasive misunderstanding exists about the available resources. The third and largest impediment to moving a national program through Congress has been the sticker shock that accompanies any serious effort to tackle long-term care.

In light of these challenges, aging and disability advocates were left wondering: What do you do if there is an enormous problem but the political system is unable or unwilling to address it? It was in this context that CLASS emerged on the scene promising "a new approach" to break through the gridlock.[21]

The Design of CLASS: Operating at Cross-Purposes

Buried deep within the Affordable Care Act, twenty pages detail the CLASS Act, a public long-term care insurance program that aspired to bring relief to the largest hole in America's social safety net.

Both in its statutory language and in the arguments put forth by its supporters, CLASS made four big, and seemingly irreconcilable, promises. First, premiums would be low. The standard premium for most enrollees would be just $30 a month and would be locked in upon signing up. (Commitment to this $30 figure was eventually abandoned when it became apparent that premiums would need to be multiple times higher and vary considerably based on age at enrollment.) Students and poor participants would need to pay only $5 a month in premiums. Following a five-year vesting period, enrollees would thereafter be eligible to receive a $50 to $100 daily benefit for life if they had long-term care needs.

Second, with just one minor exception, there would be no underwriting—the standard practice by which private insurance companies establish eligibility standards and premium structures based on an individual's likelihood of becoming benefit-eligible. CLASS' only eligibility requirement was that participants be "actively employed," and even this standard was minimal. Participants had to be working for only three out of the five pre-benefit-eligible years and had to earn a mere $1,120 annually during those three years.

The third big promise undergirding CLASS was that it would be self-sustaining—that is, the monthly premiums paid by program enrollees would cover all benefit payments without any outside subsidies.

Fourth, there would be no individual mandate. Unlike the controversial but actuarially essential requirement included in the Affordable Care Act that everyone carry health insurance, enrollment in CLASS would be entirely optional and voluntary.[22]

Under this design, CLASS was plagued by three key provisions operating at cross-purposes. The first was its voluntary structure; no one would be *required* to participate. The second was a lack of underwriting; nearly everyone would be *allowed* to participate. The third was fiscal self-sustainability; no outside subsidies would help support CLASS. The trouble with this design is that it presented a classic adverse selection problem: CLASS would be most appealing to individuals who knew they would qualify for benefits or anticipated that they might. Typically, adverse selection—a concern for any insurance offering—is addressed through underwriting, a process in which individuals with a higher likelihood of qualifying for benefits are charged higher premiums or denied the opportunity to enroll. An alternative way of dealing with adverse selection is to make enrollment mandatory, thereby ensuring that enough healthy people participate. Yet CLASS explicitly rejected both solutions. That meant there would be high demand from people disproportionately likely to qualify for benefits and low demand from everyone else (i.e., the healthy population whose premiums were needed to fund those benefits). This situation would initiate a self-perpetuating cycle—known as an "insurance death spiral"—in which premiums paid by enrollees would have to be continually raised to cover benefit payments to those needing assistance. The increasing premiums would, in turn, lead healthy individuals to quit participating in CLASS or deter them from signing up in the first place. Those reductions in healthy participants would trigger a need to increase premiums again. And so on.

Put simply, far too few people would be paying into the program to cover the costs of those receiving benefits. The numbers did not come close to adding up. Getting out of the death spiral and keeping the program afloat at that point would require massive government subsidies.

Yet in a counterintuitive twist rooted in the rules of the contemporary lawmaking process, this flawed program was deemed by the CBO to be the opposite of the financial liability that it was destined to become. For reasons that will be explained, the agency's all-important "scoring" process proclaimed CLASS to be the biggest deficit reducing element in the Affordable Care Act. These illusory savings carried major implications for the health reform process in that they made CLASS a critical, must-have component of the final legislative package. The irresistible appeal of CLASS wasn't because it was seen as an important step in addressing America's long-term care challenge; rather, it was because of the money it brought to the Affordable Care Act.

Policy Viability versus Political Viability

Two explanations are cited for CLASS' problematic design. Some have alleged that CLASS was a cynical smokescreen created and inserted into Obamacare for the purpose of deceiving lawmakers and the American public about the true costs of health reform. Others have assumed that it was an embarrassing mistake, a careless policy hastily slapped together at the last minute, or a naïve plan crafted by true believers who were in over their heads. Neither explanation is quite right.

CLASS certainly wasn't cooked up by the architects of the Affordable Care Act, most of whom wanted nothing to do with long-term care. Nor was it hastily conceived at the last minute. And it wasn't the work of idealists detached from reality. Rather, it was a carefully planned and remarkably adroit response to political reality and the institutional rules under which the congressional policymaking system now operates.

The small cohort of interest group advocates from the disability and aging communities who designed CLASS were driven by a passionate and heartfelt conviction—along with plenty of alarming demographic data—that the long-term care status quo is unacceptable and in urgent need of change. However, drawing on lessons learned from previous failures to enact long-term care reform, they knew they faced a Catch-22 scenario: *policy* viability was in conflict with *political* viability. That is, an economically viable policy that improved the nation's long-term care situation would fail to pass political muster for the reasons that doomed earlier efforts, and any proposal with a prayer of getting through the political process would be pitifully ineffective.

Yet CLASS' designers recognized that a workaround solution might be found that evaded the standard policy traps that had dogged long-term care since the 1960s: A program designed to run the *political* gauntlet—even one with obvious economic deficiencies—might have a chance of becoming law. In this way, CLASS represented an effort to use the contemporary rules of policymaking to get an economically unsound program on the books in an age when a viable program would not stand a chance.

In the context of long-term care's policy history, this counterintuitive approach was understandable. The goal was to get a program—any program—passed and, if need be, worry about improving or solidifying it later. Long-term care needed a foothold. Once that enormous barrier to entry had been achieved, supporters hoped any problems with the program could be addressed under the protection afforded by its status as law. If CLASS managed to become the law of the land, the burden would then shift from those seeking to enact a long-term care program to those seeking to repeal it.

The program's peculiarities, then, stemmed not from an overdose of idealistic naiveté or sinister Machiavellian scheming. Rather, it was a product of a sophisticated legislative strategy grounded in the lessons of past failures and dedicated to doing whatever was necessary to get a program through Congress. What CLASS offered was the possibility of an opening for achieving a national program on behalf of this unjustly marginalized policy area—and the potential for future expansion—that long-term care advocates had been chasing for decades. The key to moving CLASS through the lawmaking process did not lie in crafting a policy that might actually work; instead, it required putting forward a policy that was politically viable.

To that end, the advocates had two key insights. The first was that the "score," or cost estimate, CLASS received from the CBO would be essential to achieving political viability. The advocates knew their program would eventually have to be analyzed by the CBO, and they recognized that if they could somehow find a way for it to avoid the appearance of being a drain on the federal Treasury, that would allow CLASS to evade the exorbitant price tags that had torpedoed previous attempts to address long-term care. It would be even better if CLASS' score from the CBO showed savings. Indeed, if it was judged a money maker, CLASS would be appealing as an add-on for a larger bill because the "savings" could help pay for the larger package.

The second key insight was that the basic aspects of the CBO scoring process for proposed programs like CLASS and the Affordable Care Act are relatively transparent and therefore easy to manipulate. When estimating the cost of such programs, the CBO looks ten years into the future. This period is known as the "ten-year window." The rationale for projecting a decade into the future is that such a range represents a sweet spot: It is far enough out to get a sense for the long-term implications of a proposed program, but not so distant that one is overwhelmed by unknown factors. As a former employee of the agency explained, "CBO is governed by these rules and has to abide by them."[24] CLASS' most important design feature was the five-year vesting period in which program enrollees would pay premiums but would not be eligible to receive benefits. While waiting periods prior to benefits kicking in are common in the private long-term care insurance market, they are measured in days rather than years, and they rarely exceed 100 days.[25] The five-year waiting period for CLASS meant that when the CBO scored it, half of the ten-year scoring window would consist of the atypical period in which the program was taking in money but not paying out any benefits. And while benefit payments would commence in year six, a healthy stockpile of cash would have accumulated over the first five years. These funds would be quickly depleted once CLASS was fully operational with money coming in and going out, but the well wouldn't run dry until after the CBO's ten-year scoring window had closed.

In accordance with its standard operating procedures, and despite CLASS' clear design flaws, the CBO dutifully reported that the program would generate tens of billions of dollars in savings. Of course, those reported savings obscured the fact that once it was fully up and running it would quickly be transformed into a money pit. Notably, the CBO was not fooled. On the contrary, this critical piece of information was highlighted in the agency's analysis. The CBO clearly stated that CLASS "would add to future federal budget deficits in a large and growing fashion beginning a few years beyond the 10-year budget window."[26] But disclaimers of this sort are essentially ignored in the contemporary policymaking process. What really matters is the single price tag outputted by the CBO. One congressional staffer explained it in blunt terms: "CBO's job isn't to decide if something works, just to spit out numbers."[27]

The number that got spit out for CLASS was a big one. So big, in fact, that when CLASS was embedded in health reform, it brought along the most coveted of gifts to the larger Obama initiative: a windfall of money that would be counted as savings for the Affordable Care Act. This demonstration of savings was critical for health reform's viability because the White House and congressional Democrats had made a public commitment to deficit neutrality. In fact, the Affordable Care Act's savings constituted a key talking point for its supporters. During the public debate over health reform, President Obama even boasted that it would be "the largest deficit reduction plan in over a decade."[28] In accounting for over half of the Affordable Care Act's projected savings, CLASS was by far the biggest of these purported deficit reduction measures.

CLASS IN CONTEXT: POLICYMAKING
THROUGH LEARNING AND POLICY FAILURE

The place of the CLASS Act in long-term care's policy history and its path into the Affordable Care Act can be better understood with reference to the political science literature on the role that "learning" plays in the policymaking process. In the broadest sense, learning can be thought of as a change in beliefs based on experience and improved understanding. Policy scholars have advanced slightly different terms and conceptual frameworks for learning, including "policy learning," "social learning," "policy legacies," "lesson drawing," and "political learning."[29] Yet central to all of this work is the straightforward assertion that models purporting to explain policymaking events are misleadingly simplistic if they restrict themselves to merely considering the immediate political, interpersonal, and institutional contexts in which such events occurred.[30] Such ahistorical formulations ignore the critical role of previous debates, actions, and implementations that often set the terms for future policymaking episodes.

Peter J. May identifies a key distinction between policy learning and political learning that is useful for thinking about how failed reform efforts might lead to an important learning process. In this formulation, *policy* learning concerns the *content of policy*—"problems, goals, instruments, and implementation designs."[31] By contrast, *political* learning deals with developing more sophisticated *advocacy strategies* that are suitable for the features of a given political or policy regime. This occurs through the adoption of new political and rhetorical tactics or through expanding a coalition. In this form of learning, advocacy groups, policy experts, and lawmakers gain insights into the political costs, opportunity costs, and chances of success that different approaches offer.[32]

Most of the scholarship in social policy and health policy related to learning has been concerned with feedback effects, meaning the process by which established policies shape future policy choices by altering the capacities, interests, and beliefs of political elites and the public.[33] This work encompasses "policy failure," but generally only in the context of implemented policies that, when confronted with empirical evidence, are deemed to be failures.[34] The learning process accompanying the *failure to enact* policy proposals has not received adequate attention, though it too carries the potential to spur learning that influences future policymaking efforts.[35]

The policy and political learning approach offers a promising framework for understanding CLASS. Interest group advocates, policy experts, and lawmakers attentive to long-term care issues certainly maintain that the current system is inadequate. In that sense, their process of learning through failure is typical of the process in which established policies are exposed as inadequate or otherwise undesirable. But a different process of learning through failure carried much more influence in the development of the CLASS Act. The legacies of failed efforts to enact a national long-term care program helps explain both how CLASS succeeded in making it into the Affordable Care Act and why it was designed as it was.

Studies of policy failure can reveal key insights into how government actually works in practice. For instance, Richard E. Neustadt and Harvey V. Fineberg's classic study of the disastrous and short-lived National Influenza Immunization Program highlighted the "shaky" foundations on which many government-sponsored health initiatives rest, particularly those undertaken hastily and in response to panic and fear. Similarly, Jeffrey L. Pressman and Aaron Wildavsky's landmark examination of the Economic Development Administration's Oakland Project—a failed $23 million federal-local scheme to boost minority employment in the East Bay—illuminated the daunting practical challenges inherent in implementing detached, theoretically grounded policy. Finally, Sven Steinmo and Jon Watts emphasized the importance of institutional structure as an explanation for the repeated failures over several presidential administrations to pass comprehensive national health insurance despite a public that desired such reform.[36]

In the tradition of these policy failures, the CLASS Act carries important insights into how government really works in the twenty-first century. After decades of unsuccessful attempts to address long-term care, the designers of CLASS drew key lessons from previous failed reform efforts. The most important of these were that CLASS had to be financially self-sustaining and it could not require people to participate. By designing a program around these constraints, CLASS was able to evade the litany of roadblocks that stifled earlier proposals for a national long-term care program. Yet these very lessons gleaned from past failures—lessons that informed the creation of a politically viable proposal—also led the designers of CLASS to create a fatally flawed program.

THE NEW POLITICS OF POLICYMAKING

While the CLASS saga offers an extraordinary view of the new politics of policymaking in action, it is far from an anomaly. The tendency for the new reform-based rules to perversely shape policy is now baked into the system. And though CLASS and the Affordable Care Act were Democratic proposals, the new politics of policymaking is most certainly a bipartisan game. As chapter 7 reveals, Republicans play by the same rules.

This study analyzes the CLASS Act to gain insight into the contemporary policymaking process in Congress. Chapter 2 addresses the old system of policymaking in Washington, details the unraveling of that system amidst tensions over the budget, and then outlines the key good government reforms that were put in place to repair a process that was seen as easy to manipulate and lacking in fiscal restraint. The next four chapters present a case study of the CLASS Act that serves to highlight the pathologies and perverse incentives of the new and supposedly improved system. Chapter 3 explores several earlier attempts to establish a national long-term care program and the lessons that those unsuccessful campaigns carried for CLASS. Chapter 4 shows how a small cohort of interest group advocates working out of Ted Kennedy's Senate office learned from those failures and put together a long-shot policy proposal designed to run the gauntlet created by Washington's new rules of policymaking. Chapters 5 and 6 detail the frenzied twists and turns on Capitol Hill that saw that flawed program get inserted into—and play an important role in passing—the Affordable Care Act. Chapter 7 explores other instances of marquee legislation being shaped by the same institutional rules that informed CLASS. Finally, Chapter 8 draws conclusions about the lessons CLASS holds for today's policymaking process and for America's developing long-term care crisis. This study is partly based on dozens of extensive interviews with congressional staffers, interest group advocates, officials from the executive branch, and health policy experts. Because many of these individuals continue to work in government and because CLASS was a heated political issue with an uncertain future at the time of those discussions, most interviews were conducted with assurances that identities and affiliations would be held confidential.[37] Other primary source materials informing this study include publicly available transcripts of congressional committee hearings and floor debates, actuarial assessments, correspondence, and government documents.

Ultimately, the rise and fall of the CLASS Act contains important insights for understanding the new politics of policymaking in Washington. By opening up the legislative sausage factory, we can better understand how and why Congress creates and passes unsound public policy. The CLASS case highlights the way in which the carefully designed safeguards to prevent bad policy enshrined in the American political system can actually help incentivize the creation of the very thing they are supposed to prevent. The CLASS Act was a fundamentally flawed and unworkable policy, but one that was amazingly effective at responding to the institutional structure put in place by Congress' good government reforms. In understanding how and why an unsound policy like CLASS gets made and passed, we can gain valuable insights into how good policy might be created.

Washington's Old and New Systems of Policymaking

The "power over the purse," James Madison wrote in Federalist 58, is "the most complete and effectual weapon with which any constitution can arm the immediate representatives of the people, for obtaining a redress of every grievance, and for carrying into effect every just and salutary measure."[1] Influenced by their knowledge of conflicts between Parliament and the British Crown as well as their own experience living under the king, Madison and his fellow framers explicitly gave the legislative branch the power to tax and spend. The power of the purse provides the fuel for government activity, and it is ultimately the job of Congress to determine which activities get funded and at what level. But while the text of the Constitution may be straightforward in privileging the legislature on budgetary matters, in practice the process of shaping the nation's taxing and spending has been a joint—and often acrimonious—venture between Congress and the president, who sits atop the administrative agencies the legislative branch is asked to fund.

It should be no surprise that the budget has been a source of tension between the two branches. After all, the budget represents the high stakes table of American politics. That is because beneath all the arcane, technical verbiage, federal taxing and spending defines what government does as well as the relationship between the state and the citizen. The enduring question about what role government should play in society is fought on this battlefield. It is the budget that determines national priorities and "who gets what, when, and how."[2] Thus, what many Americans instinctively regard as an impenetrable, data-laden area of legislative affairs, determining how money is procured for the federal Treasury and how it gets spent has done more than anything else to forge the country's partisan and ideological divisions. It has historically been, and continues to be, the animating force behind much of America's political rancor.

Passage of the Congressional Budget and Impoundment Control Act of 1974 marked a watershed moment in this ongoing struggle, and its influence reached well beyond the annual budget process. The ripple effects of this reform have shaped the contemporary policymaking process in fundamental respects, and they played an important role in the development of the CLASS Act and the Affordable Care Act.[3]

It is necessary at this point to distinguish between two related governmental activities: budgeting and policymaking. The annual budget process refers to the collection of tax revenue coming into the federal Treasury and decisions concerning the appropriations, or spending, that government will undertake in the next fiscal year in support of federal programs that are already in existence. By contrast, the policymaking process refers to the many proposals for new programs that Congress considers each session as additions to the government's portfolio.

This chapter is ultimately concerned with how and why the current rules of the game for the policymaking process were established. But understanding today's policymaking process requires an appreciation of the budget process and its postwar history. Because the budget process was deemed broken, reforms were undertaken with an aim of imposing restraint. These reforms also carried important implications for the policymaking process. As such, it is necessary to understand how the budget process operated prior to the 1974 reforms, the dramatic increase in the scope of governmental activity that occurred in the 1960s, the "Budget War" following that change, and the transformational reforms that served as a peace treaty. The thing that tied these stories together was the widespread view that government spending had become reckless and out of the control by the early 1970s. This perception had developed relatively quickly, coming on the heels of decades of fiscal stability interrupted only during national crises like World War II.

Unfortunately, the well-intentioned reforms may have actually made matters worse. The new rules have failed to restrain government spending or make the budget process more transparent to the average citizen. To be sure, the reforms have altered Congress' behavior. Yet instead of instilling order, they have often led to chaos. Of particular note, the reforms created new rules aimed at establishing fiscal responsibility for those seeking to create new government programs. But in an ironic twist, these very rules created an incentive structure that encourages—or even compels—policymakers to manipulate their proposals to conform to the arbitrary standards of the new system.

PRE-REFORM BUDGETING AND ITS CRITICS

Prior to 1974, Congress had no formalized budget process at all. Instead, an informal, complex, and counterintuitive standard operating procedure prevailed. The pre-reform process of determining how to spend public funds was characterized by many relatively small spending decisions made in silos without any sense of how those expenditures fit together into an overall spending program. Some thirty-three congressional committees and subcommittees proposed funding levels for the programs under their purview. The House and Senate Appropriations panels—two of Congress' "money committees"—then determined the extent to which each of these recommendations would be funded. The House Appropriations Committee played the most important role because it acted first—almost always by appropriating less than requested. Decisions were effectively made at the subcommittee level. And while it technically would have been possible for any member of the full Appropriations Committee to take issue with a subcommittee's determinations even if he or she did not serve on that subcommittee, this virtually never occurred because a strong tradition of deference to subcommittee recommendations prevailed on the grounds that members of the subcommittee were the experts on those issues under their purview.[4]

Not surprisingly, critics alleged that making the government's spending decisions through such a fragmented process was madness. This criticism was particularly resonant among those with populist sensibilities. From the perspective of a family or small business, it does indeed seem irrational to make each spending decision in isolation and without any consideration of other expenditures. For the head of a household or a small business owner, a major financial commitment—such as buying a new car or hiring new employees—would most certainly be considered with reference to other potential outlays.

Another oddity of the pre-reform system was that the appropriations process as a whole was conducted in total isolation from any consideration of federal revenue. Instead, taxing was presided over by the other two "money committees" in Congress: House Ways and Means and Senate Finance.

This wall of separation between money coming in and money going out struck many observers as baffling and problematic. Once again, this complaint had a natural appeal, particularly to those not well versed in the ways of Capitol Hill. After all, no household or business would make spending decisions irrespective of assets and income.

This budget-making system produced a litany of would-be reformers bemoaning what appeared to be an irrational and opaque system dedicated to satisfying numerous narrow interests rather than the general interest.[5] Critics viewed the budget as merely a conglomeration of independent, disconnected parts. While these voices emerged from across the ideological spectrum, they shared a conviction that more coordination and centralization should be in place; that the process should be guided by overall national priorities; and that some mechanism should be created for considering the budget as a whole. In addition to these broad themes, liberal critics decried the disproportionate power wielded by conservative Southern Democrats who chaired the key "juice" committees, Congress' relative weakness vis-à-vis the presidency, and the secrecy of the budget process. Conservatives, meanwhile, tended to lament the system's inefficiencies, its propensity to spend increasing amounts of taxpayer money, and its habitual budget deficits.[6] While critics were abundant, the opposition to this fragmented system was itself fragmented even as the 1960s increased pressure on the federal budget and saw a sharp rise in annual deficits (as is discussed later in this chapter). The disgruntled but disorganized critics lacked a galvanizing issue or event that could bring them together.

Richard Nixon would soon provide one.

"Coordination without a Coordinator": The Hidden Virtues of the Pre-reform System

Despite hard-wired irrationalities and a growing army of detractors, America's pre-reform budgeting system worked surprisingly well. Between 1947 and 1957, there were six surpluses and five modest deficits. Adjusted for inflation and in today's dollars, the average year during this stretch saw a $13.2 billion surplus. While the subsequent decade only saw one surplus, the deficits remained remarkably small and the annual budget deficit averaged $34 billion in today's dollars. Of course, the uninitiated observer could be excused for concluding that this tally from 1947 to 1967—seven surpluses and fourteen deficits—was not particularly impressive. But in the context of federal budgeting, and particularly in light of the staggering deficits that followed, the pre-reform era running through the mid-1960s stands out as something of a golden age. By way of comparison, the decade stretching from 1975 to 1984 saw a deficit every year with an average budget that was $233.7 billion in the red (again, in today's dollars). More recently, from 2004 through 2013 there has been an inflation-adjusted deficit every year averaging $733.3 billion.[7]

How was Congress able to manage its fiscal affairs effectively through the mid-1960s, despite those institutional rules and customs that might have been expected to produce chaos?

One reason was the post-war economic boom. With revenue pouring into the Treasury, it was relatively easy to avoid making difficult choices between funding priorities. In most years, Congress was able to give competing interests larger appropriations.[8]

But congressional and budget scholars also point to another crucial factor: the distinctive features of the House money committees. Political scientist David Mayhew dubbed House Appropriations and Ways and Means "control committees," pointing out that Congress depended on them to uphold the integrity of the institution.[9] Unlike other committees that could be viewed uncharitably as forums geared toward providing their members with helpful talking points for reelection campaigns, in Appropriations and Ways and Means, the responsible grown-ups presided. They ensured that the particular interests of individual representatives and interest group pressure did not destroy the institutional integrity of the House or completely undermine the common good. A key role for Ways and Means and Appropriations, then, was to take on the necessary but difficult tasks that most members of Congress—who were too busy wooing their constituents—wanted to avoid. In deference to this vital but potentially burdensome role, control committees enjoyed special rules, both formal and informal, that insulated them from outside pressures. For instance, there was a norm of appointing moderates to Appropriations and Ways and Means, and both panels had a strong nonpartisan culture. Additionally, when legislation from Ways and Means went to the House floor, "the closed rule" prohibited amendments, thereby acting "as a shield . . . against hundreds of interest group demands."[10]

The unique roles of House Appropriations and Ways and Means also helped engender fiscal responsibility. Appropriations played the role of "the sheriff warding off the mob" and "guardian of the federal Treasury" by approaching budget requests with skepticism and looking to trim budgets at every turn.[11] Committee members—liberals and conservatives alike—were unusually unified in their shared commitment for cutting spending and reducing budgets. The longer one served on the committee, the more entrenched this mindset became.[12] Ways and Means also took seriously its responsibility to safeguard the nation's well-being and the institutional integrity of the full House of Representatives. Chairman Wilbur Mills (D-AR), who prominently presided over the committee from 1958 to 1974, would say that as a matter of practice, these grave responsibilities meant that "this committee must always proceed with the utmost caution, responsibility, and prudence."[13] Like most Ways and Means members, Mills was dedicated to protecting the influence and prestige the committee enjoyed. He thought the best way to maintain that privileged position was to ensure that all legislation put out by Ways and Means was economically sound and likely to be passed on the House floor. These tasks could be achieved by crafting legislation with great care and by fostering compromise.[14] As one Ways and Means member emphasized during the Mills era, "We always try for a consensus. [Other committees] battle it out."[15]

The Ways and Means Committee's dedication to responsibility was particularly on display in its efforts to balance the short-term, constituent-specific goals that typify Congress' activities with higher objectives like maintaining sufficient revenues to fund government spending.[16] Its approach to Social Security offers an illustrative example. During the 1950s and 1960s, pressure to liberalize benefits was substantial, and the Senate Finance Committee was eager to embrace this politically popular impulse. But expanding benefits threatened to undermine the program's fiscal solvency and stability. Martha Derthick's classic study of Social Security concluded that "[p]erhaps the most important function of the legislative committees was to reconcile the legislature's conflicting impulses and strike a balance between benefits and revenues. For this purpose, the Ways and Means Committee enforced a norm of 'fiscal soundness' that was absolutely central." This meant guarding the program's actuarial soundness and keeping the tax burden within reasonable limits by extending benefits slowly. Thus, Ways and Means played the role of restraining the program's expansion until financing was secured to pay for it. The result was that Social Security expanded more slowly and incrementally than some wanted. But when expansion did occur, it was based on a more solid foundation than it otherwise would have been, and that helped reinforce the program's economic and political stability.[17]

In sum, the old system of budgeting worked fairly well despite its eccentric features. To be sure, the postwar economic boom helped

mightily by producing a steady flow of revenue. But it was also facil-
itated by the unique roles, responsibilities, and norms of the money
committees in the House. Their job was to maintain "actuarial soundness," demand "fiscal responsibility," "ward off ... real dangers," and
generally act as brakemen "on what can all too easily become a runaway engine."[18] Perhaps most importantly, the restraint and responsibility that characterized Appropriations and Ways and Means helped
to keep the nation's fiscal sheet balanced, maintain sound social programs, and consistently produce either surpluses or minor deficits in
the postwar era.

The leading scholar of the budget process, Aaron Wildavsky, recognized that this pre-reform system possessed a number of strengths. He
concluded that it was an "idyllic" and "marvelous example of coordination without a coordinator."[19] Despite being decentralized and "bottom-
up" in operation, it managed to produce cohesive and orderly results. The
process was timely; spending was roughly on par with tax revenue; it sim-
plified a very complex task into many manageable decisions; it avoided
noticeable economic problems or significant political conflict; it facili-
tated compromise, an essential feature of democratic governance; and
it was a system that—for most of its life, anyway—was generally seen as
legitimate. For Wildavsky, that was a lot to admire. Sure, it might be possible to improve the system in certain respects, but Wildavsky cautioned
that the grand and idealistic reforms most commonly bandied about on
both the ideological right and left were naïve and would "turn out to be
unfeasible, undesirable, or both." Ultimately, he argued, the budgetary
process and America's political system were inextricably linked. "The tradition of reform in America is a noble one," he wrote. "But in this case it
is doomed to failure because it is aimed at the wrong target. If the present
budgetary process is rightly or wrongly deemed unsatisfactory, then one
must alter in some respect the political system of which the budget is but
an expression."[20] By 1974, however, the old system's perceived legitimacy
had suffered considerably, and Wildavsky and its other defenders were
clearly on the defensive.

"YEAH, BUT I'LL TAKE CARE OF THAT": A POLICYMAKING EPISODE IN THE PRE-REFORM ERA

At the same time that the budgeting system was under assault, new cracks were developing in the policymaking process. President Lyndon Johnson's approach to passing Medicare in 1965 offers a classic example of how the old system of policymaking could be abused. The national social insurance program for senior citizens was a crowning achievement of Johnson's presidency and the centerpiece of his "Great Society." But pursuing that highbrow agenda required the kind of old-fashioned, whatever-it-takes politics for which LBJ was famous. Other presidents—notably Harry Truman and John Kennedy—had tried and failed to overhaul American health care. Johnson thought those setbacks had occurred because Congress always got cold feet when confronted with cost projections for a new program. In his memoir, Johnson wrote: "The Ways and Means Committee had been the graveyard" for previous Medicare proposals because Chairman Mills "was a man who stood on principle—and on principle he was worried about the 'actuarial soundness' of the administration's plan to finance Medicare."[21]

To avoid his predecessors' fates, Johnson misrepresented Medicare's costs and leaned on his allies in Congress to rush the bill through the lawmaking process. As scholars David Blumenthal and James Morone have shown, he deliberately lowballed the program's long-term economic impact and attempted to suppress projections of Medicare's real costs from becoming public.[22] (He similarly concealed news that the Vietnam War was escalating as was the cost of fighting it, knowing such information would lead Congress and the public to question the viability of paying for "guns and butter" at the same time.[23])

In an illustrative phone call between Johnson and Mills, for instance, Johnson insisted that he had already taken care of the fiscal issues. When the Ways and Means chairman expressed the misgiving LBJ anticipated— Medicare cost too much and did not fit the budget—Johnson blithely dismissed the concern, explaining that his own frugal budgeting meant extra money was available: "Yeah, but I'll take care of that. I'll do that. You see what I've done, Wilbur, ... by constant Cabinet pressure, by withholding, and just threatening, and ultimatum, and being meaner than you or [Senate Finance Committee Chair] Harry Byrd [D-VA], I am under [budget] this year ... a billion, eight hundred million under what [Congress] appropriated and what I said I'd spend."[24]

Johnson's explanation failed to make clear how coming in under budget in 1965 would help fund Medicare for decades to come, but Mills did not have a chance to ask follow-up questions because the president transitioned into a blanket dismissal of cost concerns in deference to the greater good. In this instance he launched into a story that disparaged the very concept of cost concerns:

> When they asked me: "Do you want to put in $400 or $500 million [in additional annual costs to pay for a larger Medicare program than initially proposed]?" ... What did I say about it? ... I said, well you tell Wilbur [Mills] we had an old judge in Texas one time, we called him Alcalde. Old Alcalde Roberts. And he said, when they [accused] him one time that he might've abused the Constitution, and he said, "Well, what's the Constitution between friends?" And I say, tell Wilbur that $400 million's not going to separate us friends when it's for health.[25]

Likewise, in discussing the matter with House Speaker John McCormack (D-MA), Johnson noted: "You know my philosophy, and yours: You and I never argued about $450 million for people over 65, did we?"[26] For Johnson, Medicare was worth whatever it cost.

But while LBJ might have been willing to pay any price, he knew others would be more frugal. Moreover, Medicare was also facing opposition for a number of other reasons, including physicians' fear of government control. So Johnson leaned on his congressional allies to rush the program through the lawmaking process before potential opponents had the chance to "generate opposition to us." In this effort, he had big advantages. The opposition was unaware of what exactly would be included in the Medicare bill Johnson and Mills were putting together or when it might be released. In a phone call with advisor Wilbur Cohen, Johnson said: "Now, tell the Speaker and Wilbur [Mills] to [move the legislation quickly and] not to let it lay around. Do that. They want to [do it quickly], but they might not. Then that gets . . . the others organized. . . . It stinks. It's just like a dead cat on the door. When a committee reports it, you better either bury that cat or get some life into it." Having found a metaphor he was pleased with, Johnson employed it directly to congressional leaders, too. To Mills, he said: "Now, for God's sake don't let the dead cat stand on your porch . . . when you get [the bill] out of that committee, you call that son of a bitch up before they can get their letters written."[27]

Johnson's strategy was largely effective. Only when the executive branch's Bureau of the Budget (without prior authorization from the White House) tallied up the numbers and announced an estimate did Johnson have to back away from including certain types of coverage in Medicare. In being forced to accept these modest changes, he expressed indignation that anyone would question his program or do the math to figure out how much it would cost. During a call with Senator Edward Kennedy (D-MA), Johnson angrily explained his frustration with the cost projections and what he saw as the predictable hysteria they caused: "The fools [at the Bureau of the Budget] had to go projecting [Medicare] down the road five or six years. And . . . first thing, [Senator] Dick Russell [D-GA] comes running in saying, 'My God, you've got a one billion dollar [projection] for next year on health; therefore, I'm against any of it now.' Do you follow me?"[28]

While Johnson may not have gotten everything he wanted, he did get a much more expansive law than would otherwise have passed Congress. And in this case, of course, many would conclude that whatever obfuscation Johnson employed in pursuit of Medicare was well worth it. After all, the program quickly established itself as a sacred pillar of America's social safety net, and it remains popular today.

Nonetheless, LBJ's manipulations and dismissal of legitimate budgetary questions revealed a system that could be easily gamed by those in positions of power or with the kind of political skill—that is, bullying— embodied by the infamous "Johnson treatment." Indeed, some future leader might take advantage of the weaknesses in the system and exploit them for less sanguine purposes.

THE DEVELOPMENT OF THE WELFARE STATE

Medicare's addition to the welfare state was a key step in a gradual shift in government's role in American society. This change put pressure on and eventually fractured the stability of the pre-reform budget system. Following the postwar boom, federal spending had increased dramatically and well in excess of revenues. In the twenty years prior to the 1974 reforms, annual federal expenditures had more than tripled, and only one surplus had been registered since 1960. While the deficits were initially modest, they were trending upward and saw an alarmingly sharp increase in the late 1960s and early 1970s.[29]

The development of the American welfare state was the most significant and enduring force behind the federal government's inability to control spending. Though the United States is often described as a comparative "laggard" in its welfare state provisions, it undertook significant social commitments during the presidencies of Democrats Franklin Roosevelt and Lyndon Johnson. The Social Security Act, which established a public pension system and a number of welfare programs, constituted the linchpin of FDR's New Deal expansion in the 1930s. LBJ's Great Society additions were anchored by two major health programs, the aforementioned Medicare (for the old) and Medicaid (primarily for the poor). Once these new programs were fully operational, they drastically increased federal spending. From 1965 (before Great Society spending) to 1973 (following full implementation), nondefense domestic spending increased from 9.9 to 13.2 percent of gross national product, and more than half of this jump stemmed from the Great Society programs.[30] These latter expansions were effectively ratified by Johnson's successor, Republican Richard Nixon, who chose to not only refrain from challenging his predecessor's accomplishments, but to expand the welfare state further. With support from the Nixon administration, federal spending again increased dramatically in

1972 with a 20 percent boost in Social Security benefits and the creation of new programs for higher education and the states that cost tens of billions of dollars. Taken cumulatively, these transformations in the scope of government activity meant that by the early 1970s, millions of American families were receiving substantial public support under massive programs endorsed by both major political parties.[31]

This expanded American welfare state brought what budget scholar Allen Schick called "a radical change in the composition of the federal budget."[32] Understanding the implications of this change requires an appreciation of the key distinction between "discretionary" and "mandatory" expenditures. Traditionally, discretionary spending has been the norm, and it continues to be the type of spending that pays for most things that the government actually does, from national defense to fighting forest fires to maintaining the interstate highway system. This type of spending is dubbed "discretionary" because it is up to the discretion of the appropriations committees to determine every year how much money will be spent on each budget item. Typically, the committees make these decisions based on their assessments of national priorities, the current state of the economy, and the requested budgets from each governmental unit (for example, the Department of Defense, the Department of Agriculture, and so on). As discussed earlier, in the pre-reform era, the House Appropriations Committee operated under the assumption that most spending requests were inflated beyond what was necessary, and committee members saw it as their job to exercise discretion by reducing spending below the requested levels. A key point here is that discretionary spending allows great flexibility for the appropriations committees in Congress to determine how much money is spent and what it is spent on.

Mandatory spending is different in the critical respect that Congress lacks the spending flexibility it enjoys with discretionary outlays. The overwhelming majority of mandatory spending goes to the big three "entitlement" programs: Social Security, Medicare, and Medicaid.[33] In these areas, the government is legally required to provide benefits to all qualified individuals. This means that if fifty million Americans meet the eligibility requirements for Medicare, the government is legally obligated to provide each of them with the full menu of benefits that had been promised to them, regardless of other spending priorities or the state of the economy. The appropriations committees have no oversight role, nor do they have the authority to adjust this type of spending. Thus, one consequence of each expansion of government-sponsored social provisions funded through mandatory spending was that the appropriations committees lost some control over federal spending.

Since the early 1960s, mandatory spending has consumed an ever larger share of the federal budget. In the early 1960s, about 30 percent of it consisted of mandatory spending. By 1974—the year of major budget reforms and nearly a decade after the enactment of Medicare and Medicaid—this figure had shot up to 49 percent. In fiscal year 2012, nearly 64 percent of the federal budget went to mandatory programs, with entitlement spending alone accounting for more than 57 percent of the entire budget. Looking at it from a slightly different angle, and adjusting for inflation and population growth, in 2010 the United States spent almost seven times more on entitlements than it did in 1960. Meanwhile, national defense— which has consumed over half of all discretionary spending each year since the Iraq War—comprised 20 percent of the total budget pie. All told, well over half of the annual federal budget now goes to pay for entitlement programs while only 17 percent goes to nondefense discretionary spending.[34] Projections indicate this trend of increasing mandatory spending and decreasing discretionary spending will continue.

Today, observers spanning the ideological spectrum are concerned about this trajectory. A general anxiety is that current spending and future commitments are unsustainable and have placed the country on an untenable fiscal path. This view, for instance, served as the jumping off point for the bipartisan Simpson Bowles Commission created by President Obama in 2010.[35] Many on the political right also allege that traditional American values such as independence, self-reliance, and hard work have been replaced by a culture of dependence.[36] Meanwhile, those on the left worry that unceasing increases in mandatory spending will "crowd out" spending for other vital services performed by government. For example, Will Marshall of the Progressive Policy Institute notes that "the big entitlement programs . . . squeeze out public investment" in critical non-entitlement areas:

> [D]omestic spending supports priorities liberals once fought and bled for. These include common goods like transport, water, and other vital infrastructure that supports economic growth; our national commitment to science and technology[;] and, the public education and training institutions that make "equal opportunity" more than a hollow slogan. Also being starved are progressive programs to help people lift themselves out of poverty, curb hunger, and expand early learning opportunities for families that can't afford costly day care, not to mention environmental protection, public health and law enforcement.[37]

These contemporary concerns are not new; they've been prevalent since the early 1970s. As bills came due for President Johnson's Great Society programs and the war in Vietnam, it appeared that the government was simply in the habit of chronically running budget deficits.[38] The spike in budget deficits caused widespread concern that federal spending was "out of control" and needed to be addressed. Yet the expansion of the welfare state changed the nature of what American government did and the way in which Congress behaved. New entitlements upended the institutional norms that once kept a lid on spending, and Congress' ability to control federal spending was substantially weakened. As the newly expanded welfare state operated and spent money outside the purview of the regular appropriations process, the scope of activity for the appropriations committees decreased, and the flexibility Congress enjoyed in the realm of discretionary spending was greatly curtailed.[39] The result was an altered budget system in which spending and deficits were skyrocketing, and the restraining features of the old system were no longer able to exert their customary influence. The genie was out of the bottle.

REFORMS IN PURSUIT OF DISCIPLINE AND RESPONSIBILITY

Out of this basic problem—uncontrollable spending that far exceeded revenue—other related reasons for reform sprang up, the most prominent of which was a bitter feud between the legislative and executive branches during the Nixon presidency.[40] A decline in trust between the branches predated Nixon's ascension to the White House. Congress had traditionally relied on the executive branch's Office of Management and Budget (known as the Bureau of the Budget until 1970) for budget estimates and economic forecasting. The agency had long maintained a sterling reputation for independence and reliability, but that luster had been tarnished during the Johnson and Nixon administrations when the agency had come to be seen as part of the president's political operation.[41] From Congress' perspective, the executive branch was no longer a trustworthy supplier of data and analysis. Meanwhile, facing a fiscally troubled federal government and a Congress under Democratic control, Nixon became more confrontational.

Nixon campaigned for reelection in 1972 on the budget issue and found a good culprit to implicate. He denounced the "accidental, haphazard" approach taken by Congress to budgeting and the "unbridled increases in Federal spending." "At fault," he charged, "is the hoary and traditional procedure of the Congress, which now permits action on the various spending programs as if they were unrelated and independent." Of course, the budget system the president denounced had worked well prior to the massive expansion of the welfare state in the 1960s and early 1970s—a process in which Nixon himself had played a significant role. Nonetheless, the counterintuitive and opaque budgeting process employed by Congress made for a better villain than popular social programs. It shouldn't be a surprise, then, that once budget pressures mounted, Nixon joined the herd in singling out the budget system to take the blame. Nixon warned that "[w]ith or without the cooperation of Congress, I am going to do everything within my power to prevent such a fiscal crisis."[42]

Following a landslide reelection victory, Nixon acted on his threat and began "impounding"—or refusing to spend—funds appropriated by

Congress. This aggressive action marked the peak of the so-called Budget War.[43] There was historical precedent for this action, though Nixon's use of impoundments differed in an important way. Many presidents had previously impounded funds that were deemed no longer necessary. Thomas Jefferson, for instance, impounded $50,000 in congressionally appropriated funds that were to be used for the purchase of gunboats to patrol the Mississippi River. But following a peaceful "turn of affairs," he judged the outlay to be unnecessary. Nixon's impoundments differed in that they were not narrowly employed to avoid needless expenditures born of unforeseen circumstance. Instead, Nixon used impoundments as a "political weapon" with the goal of reducing or defunding programs he opposed.[44] Many members of Congress reacted in horror and accused the president of unconstitutionally undermining the separation of powers and Congress' power of the purse.

The impoundment dispute was directly related to the nation's fiscal problems. As one budget scholar explained, "it is exceedingly difficult to separate the impact of the incredibly troublesome economy from the growing congressional conflict with the president, except to say that the former tended to exacerbate and provide context for the latter."[45] The standoff forced Congress to realize that it had to be proactive in tackling the fiscal problems that provoked the confrontation between the branches.

The Congressional Budget and Impoundment Control Act of 1974

The Congressional Budget and Impoundment Control Act of 1974—colloquially known as the Budget Act—had ambitious aims. Lawmakers recognized that merely reasserting congressional prerogatives over the budget would be insufficient. Senator Lee Metcalf (D-MT), for instance, declared: "The plain facts are that regardless of who exercises authority, the budget is in danger of going out of control."[46] Instilling fiscal restraint was therefore critical. As articulated in the bill's language and by its supporters, the legislation was supposed to control budget deficits, limit federal spending, prioritize spending, enable Congress to compete effectively with the president on budget matters, and complete the annual budget process in a timely manner.

The law contained four important features, two of which would come to play central roles in the CLASS story. The two aspects unrelated to CLASS saw a series of procedures to reassert the power of the purse held by Congress by preventing presidents from ignoring the spending decisions made on Capitol Hill and the establishment of a new and much more formalized budget process anchored by the creation of a Budget Committee in both the House and the Senate. These new committees were intended to consider the overall picture of government finance, to operate as control mechanisms to prevent a runaway budget, and to shift more power to Capitol Hill.

More importantly for CLASS and the policymaking process in general was the creation of the Congressional Budget Office (CBO). The agency was tasked with providing budgetary information, advice, and support to Congress. It would perform these tasks in two distinct areas: the annual budget process and new policy proposals. The idea of an institution like the CBO was not new in 1974. In fact, a nearly identical governmental organization had already been operational for several decades. The Office of Management and Budget had been performing similar tasks to those that the CBO would be undertaking since 1921. But the Office of Management and Budget was part of the executive branch and was controlled by the president. By creating the CBO, Congress was asserting its independence and ensuring that it would no longer be beholden to reports and data produced at the pleasure of the president. The CBO would now offer Congress its own in-house analysis of the annual budget process and new policy proposals. And that promised to strengthen the position of Congress vis-à-vis the president.

In a remarkable and unusual move for an institution that is structured around partisanship, Congress determined that the CBO would be explicitly apolitical. After all, if this new institution was supposed to give Congress the tools it needed to impose discipline, order, and stability on the budgeting and policymaking processes, it necessarily followed that it had to be producing independent and reliable information. As one participant succinctly noted in an important organizational meeting in 1975, "[the CBO] has the task of presenting materials that will lead to rational decision making by Congress."[47] And that meant that the new agency needed to be staffed with economists and experts who earned their jobs based on training, technical expertise, and competence rather than political patronage. Today, most of the CBO's approximately 235 employees are economists or public policy analysts with graduate degrees. The agency issues between 500 and 700 cost estimates for proposed legislation each year as well as numerous other annual reports on the budget. The two houses of Congress jointly appoint the CBO's director, who, according to the Budget Act, must be selected without regard to partisan affiliation.[48] Many view the CBO as one of the few straight shooters in Washington's swamp of partisan connivers. It is a strictly empirical, nonjudgmental agency with no interest in normative debates over whether a particular bill *ought* to become law.

The final notable feature of the Budget Act that would later heavily influence both CLASS and the policymaking system more broadly is reconciliation.[49] The reconciliation process—now considered a viable means of passing legislation—was originally something of an afterthought in the Budget Act, and it had a specific and quite limited purpose. The basic point of reconciliation was to force budget retrenchment, either through lowering spending or through increasing revenue. As laid out in the 1974 law, the new annual budget process was supposed to include two budget resolutions, or measures agreed upon by both the House and the Senate to establish Congress' budget. The first of these would be enacted in May and would be a tentative projection of spending, revenue, and the budget deficit or surplus. The second budget resolution would be adopted in September, and it would be binding. Reconciliation was supposed to be a part of this second stage of the annual budget process. It was created—as the term implies—to reconcile any changes that had emerged between the first resolution in May and the second in September due to the passage of other laws that affected the budget. It was supposed to make only minor alterations and, in addressing changes that had already occurred, be backward looking in nature. With the aim of facilitating action in the new budget process—and in contrast to normal Senate procedure—debate was limited for reconciliation bills, which would not be subject to filibusters and would be allowed to pass with a simple majority vote.

Congress formally passed the Budget Act by lopsided margins (75-0 in the Senate and 401-6 in the House), and on July 12, 1974, President Nixon—who would resign less than a month later amidst the Watergate scandal—signed the bill into law. He praised Congress' efforts to address "overspending by government" and asserted that the "lack of discipline in Congressional procedures has been one of the major factors behind the sizable increases in Federal spending over the last decade.... Congress has wisely recognized these weaknesses and taken steps to correct them through the passage of this legislation."[50]

Assessing the Reforms

The 1974 Budget Act is widely considered a failure, albeit one with an important redeeming feature: the creation of the CBO. As Louis Fisher, a Library of Congress scholar, wrote in commemoration of the law's tenth anniversary: The Budget Act "has led a charmed life. Rarely has a statute missed goals by such wide margins without being repealed or severely amended."[51] While it halted presidential impoundments and created new mechanisms for Congress to independently exercise its power of the purse, the larger goal of corralling federal spending was an abject failure.[52] The reformed annual budget process has been singled-out as particularly disgraceful. Fisher, for instance, calls it "embarrassing both in operation and results."[53] Among other difficulties, it has been routinely late at each stage of the process, unable to control deficits or limit spending, unable to force lawmakers to identify budget priorities, and has become reliant on crisis budgeting crutches like last-minute omnibus spending packages and continuing resolutions under the threat of government shutdowns.[54]

Observers maintain that the law has not only been unsuccessful, but it has actually exacerbated the very problems with the budget process that it was supposed to solve. An underlying assumption of the Budget Act was that members of Congress would conduct themselves more responsibly if they were forced to grapple with the overall budget instead of voting separately on numerous appropriation packages, a process that made it difficult to grasp the full picture. That is not the way it worked out. Members of Congress quickly invented work-arounds to avoid the unpleasantness of curtailing spending or boosting revenues with new taxes. Rather than reining in spending and deficits, the reforms dramatically weakened control and incentivized the gaming of the system.[55] Representative David Obey (D-WI)—a persistent critic of the post-1974 system—observed in 1985 that "the only kind of budget resolution that can pass today is one that lies ... because you cannot get members under the existing system to face up to what the real numbers are. You always wind up having phony economic assumptions and all kinds of phony numbers on estimating."[56] Former CBO director Rudy Penner has expressed similar disenchantment. He has acknowledged that he was "one of those public policy analysts who thought the 1974 process was a good idea when it was first invented." Yet he later developed buyer's remorse. "I have to confess to a lot of disappointment and frustration as to how it actually worked out." Testifying before Congress in 1990, Penner reflected on the shakeup: "I have always been struck by the fact, in looking at the history of the process, that it appeared chaotic in the late 19th century and early 20th century, but the results were very good in terms of budget discipline, yielding balanced budgets or surpluses most of the time." The new system, by contrast, "looks very elegant on paper, but it is leading to very dishonest and disorderly results."[57]

The CBO and the Policymaking Process

According to conventional wisdom, the one shining exception to the Budget Act's legacy of disappointment is the CBO and its influential role in the policymaking process. Philip G. Joyce, a public policy scholar and former CBO employee, offers the leading account of the agency. Prior to the CBO's existence, Joyce explains, a number of nefarious schemes were employed by lawmakers and advocates to hide the true costs of their proposed policies. Among other accounting tactics, "the camel's nose strategy" relied on a slow phase-in of a program to obscure the major economic commitment its future entailed. Metaphorically, the camel represented the cost of a proposed new program. Yet within the policymaking tent, only the camel's nose—representing a very small percentage of the total camel—was visible with the rest to be recognized only after the commitment had been made and it was too late to turn back. In the face of such budgetary gimmicks, Congress decided that "[p]olicymakers and their constituents needed to be confronted with the truth—in the form of the most neutral analysis possible on budgetary and economic implications of particular policy choices." For Joyce, the insertion of this "unbiased referee" was a game changer: "The result has exceeded the wildest expectations of those who conceived and established the institution. The CBO has developed a clear and sustained reputation for counteracting the natural tendency of the political system to sugarcoat the fiscal news."[58]

The agency is perhaps at its best, according to prevailing sentiment, when it is producing cost estimates for proposed new programs. When a bill is reported out of committee, the CBO is mandated to "score" it. This process involves analyzing changes that would occur to federal outlays and revenues if the bill were implemented as written. In generating the score, the CBO projects ten years into the future and assumes that all current laws hold during that period. As noted in chapter 1, the rationale for this "ten-year window" is that it is sufficient to get a sense for the long-term implications of proposed programs but not so far into the future that one loses the ability to make reasonably informed projections. The CBO then compares the final projected cost to the "baseline" projections it makes each year in order to decide if new legislation would increase or decrease deficits. Some bills require complicated economic modeling that outside experts can contest, but the CBO score is generally viewed as an authoritative verdict on a bill's cost.

The CBO score can have important effects on legislation. First, the score affects elite and public opinion of the legislation. Although the CBO produces detailed analyses of proposed legislation, lawmakers and the public tend to focus on the numerical projection the agency makes about the proposed legislation's cost. It is taken as the gold standard on Capitol Hill and often plays a critical role in debates over bills. Unfortunately, this tendency to focus exclusively on a single number does a disservice to the CBO's careful work. As helpful and important as the single figure is, it can obscure as much as it reveals. As the CBO's former acting director Donald B. Marron cautions, "cost estimates cannot speak for themselves. There is a natural tendency to focus solely on the bottom line ... but by itself, a cumulative 10-year cost says little about the merits [or] the long-run budget impacts of particular policies."[59]

Second, the CBO score can trigger budgetary requirements in other laws. For example, the Statutory Pay-As-You-Go Act of 2010 requires that "all new legislation changing taxes, fees, or mandatory expenditures, taken together, must not increase projected deficits."[60] If Congress does pass legislation that increases deficits, in the CBO's judgment, mandatory "sequestration"—spending cuts—can automatically take effect. This and other legislative budget requirements make it extraordinarily difficult for Congress to pass new legislation that receives a high cost projection from the CBO.

The CBO is designed to counter the kind of misrepresentation used by President Johnson and his allies back in 1965. And for many, the agency has played its role to perfection. Joyce, for instance, concludes that "it would be hard to paint CBO cost estimating as anything but successful" because Congress now has what it previously lacked: "credible, multi-year estimates on the costs of proposed legislation. Moreover, Congress must pay attention to these estimates, which has the effect of introducing greater fiscal responsibility into the process."[61]

Yet despite all the benefits that come from having reliable, nonpartisan estimates for the fiscal implications of legislative proposals, the 1974 reforms that inserted the CBO into the policymaking process have produced similar problems to those encountered by the annual budget process. Proposed new programs now receive a level of scrutiny that programs from the Great Society and before did not have to face. To a large degree, this is a positive development. However, the new rules have introduced new problems as well. Two are particularly noteworthy. First, and in stark contrast to the passage of Medicare, the new system has institutionalized an obsession with the budgetary implications of proposed programs. Such concerns are, of course, entirely sensible. But it has yielded a policymaking environment in which the key issue in many policy debates now is whether a proposed program adds to or subtracts from budget deficits. Questions about the merits of, or need for, a particular program and whether that program and its costs constitute an acceptable expansion of government activity are often relegated to second-tier status if they are considered at all. The other, related problem is that as policymakers have become accustomed to the new rules of the game, they have discovered work-arounds. The CBO has introduced a process for assessing legislation that can be manipulated, and the agency's crucial role in the legislative process makes such manipulation very appealing and rewarding. With the CBO watching, Congress has two options: Either pass only fiscally responsible legislation or make laws *appear* as though they are revenue neutral or, even better, cost savers. This manipulation of a policy's appearance can allow flawed or even unworkable policies to become law.

Follow-Up Reforms: Reconciliation and the Byrd Rule

In light of disappointments over the efficacy of the Budget Act, a number of revisions and pieces of follow-up legislation were passed, and one of these additional reforms came to play an important role in the story of the CLASS Act as well as the larger Obama health-care overhaul.[62] These follow-up reforms constituted attempts to revise aspects of the 1974 law and, at their core, to deal with the same fundamental problem that spurred the Budget Act in the first place. "The Byrd Rule," a 1985 amendment to the Budget Act, was among these follow-up reforms.

During the Carter and Reagan administrations, reconciliation began to be used to pass legislation that went well beyond the scope and intent of the original process. Two changes in the use of reconciliation stood out. First, the original understanding that reconciliation was supposed to be used only for reducing deficits had been abandoned. Second, instead of using reconciliation as a backward-looking mechanism to reconcile minor changes between the first and second budget resolutions each year, the process began to be used during the first stage of the process. In effect, this change greatly expanded its potential use, and reconciliation began to be employed as a means of passing legislation that would have otherwise been stopped in the normal legislative process.

Unsettled by this greatly expanded use of reconciliation and the deviation from Senate custom that it represented, some members of the body, led by Robert Byrd (D-WV), sought to rein in these abuses by clarifying what kinds of legislation were permissible under the process. Named for its chief sponsor, the Byrd Rule was designed to protect the integrity of the reconciliation process by excluding from consideration any "extraneous matter" that failed to facilitate deficit reduction. A provision is considered "extraneous" if it does not produce a change in government revenues or if the change produced is "merely incidental." Any senator is allowed to challenge the inclusion of a provision on these grounds. Upon such a challenge, the Senate parliamentarian—an appointed official with expertise in the upper chamber's complex rules and procedures—settles the dispute. If the parliamentarian sustains a challenge then the impermissible provision is removed.[63]

Despite the Byrd Rule, ensuing years have seen reconciliation continue to be used in ways that are out of keeping with its original intention. The signature legislative accomplishments of the two most recent presidents—the Bush tax cuts and the Affordable Care Act—offer prime examples. However, whatever its shortcomings, the Byrd Rule did establish some limits to the use of reconciliation, and those limits ended up playing an important role in the final stage of the lawmaking process for the CLASS Act.

While the 1974 Budget Act succeeded in generating more information for Congress, it did not alter the inherently political nature of the system; it just created a new set of rules. And as Wildavsky cautioned, "people learn to play any system." Budgeting and policymaking are fundamentally political processes. Enlightened attempts to deny the political nature of these processes or to elevate them to a higher plane are destined to yield unintended consequences to which everyone has to adjust and take into consideration when planning a legislative strategy.[64] The long-term care crisis to which the CLASS Act was responding is impossible to deny. The advocates who designed the program had to play by the same rules as everyone else.

The rules of the policymaking game have undoubtedly changed in the fifty years since Lyndon Johnson pushed his Great Society initiatives through Congress. But the possibilities and incentives for manipulating the rules still exist. If he were alive today and placed in the middle of Washington's policymaking orbit, LBJ might even feel as if he had never left.

A Legacy of Failure

*Long-Term Care's Policy History
and the Genesis of the CLASS Act*

Long-term care has become a challenge for the United States (and many other countries) because of a positive development: We are living longer than ever. However, and without dismissing all of the great benefits associated with longer lives, the bad news is that living longer can be very expensive. The average American citizen may have little awareness of this looming problem, but it is one that policy experts have recognized for decades. The CLASS Act was the latest, but certainly not the first, attempt to find a solution. When Medicare was enacted in 1965, it was anticipated that a long-term care benefit would be added in short order. Yet in the decades that followed, this once probable addition to Medicare became marginalized. Throughout the 1970s, numerous reform proposals, many championed by Representative Claude Pepper (D-FL), sought to create a national long-term care program, but none came close to fruition. In the next two decades, long-term care had three big moments in the policy spotlight.[1] All three—the Medicare Catastrophic Coverage Act, the Pepper Commission, and the Clinton health reform effort—ended in embarrassing and high-profile failure. For most of the Washington political establishment, these debacles suggested that sweeping plans for a national long-term care program were politically untenable.

Yet for one small band of advocates and lawmakers, these failures carried a different set of political lessons that informed the CLASS Act.

"THERE ARE THINGS WHICH REMAIN TO BE DONE": MEDICARE'S ENACTMENT (1965)

During the 1965 Medicare debates in Congress, long-term care—particularly in the form of nursing home care—was part of the discussion and could have been folded into the social insurance program.[2] The issue received extensive attention in hearings before the Senate Finance Committee in which several senators proposed adding long-term care provisions. Senator Russell Long (D-LA) fought to remove coverage limitations for extended hospital stays. Going further, Senator Abraham Ribicoff (D-CT) introduced a much more extensive amendment to cover an array of long-term care services and argued that Congress "should not lose this opportunity to do the whole job."[3] Similar proposals in the House contained provisions for long-term care.[4] Ultimately, however, all these plans were left out of the final legislative package of Representative Wilbur Mills (D-AR).

At the time, the failure to provide for long-term care was recognized as a key limitation in the landmark law.[5] The *Wall Street Journal*, for instance, anticipated that "there will be widespread disappointment when old folks realize the program won't pay for ... long-term 'custodial' residence in nursing homes."[6] Meanwhile, Senator Jacob Javits (R-NY) lamented the pending Medicare bill's lack of long-term care provisions but nonetheless urged his colleagues to support the legislation: "It still will not deal with those who are chronically ill and need continuous care, but it is still a very long way in the direction of a full health care program" that Congress had been trying to make workable for so many years.[7] In a similar vein, Representative Pepper spoke in favor of the legislation despite its lack of a long-term care provision during the House floor debate: "[T]here are things which remain to be done. We do not provide in this bill for the aged chronically ill. ... I hope that will be one of the challenges of the future, and that we may find a way [so that] those who have to stay in a hospital or a nursing home for a longer period than allowed by this bill will be succored while in the period of illness and confinement."[8]

Despite the recognition that Medicare coverage contained gaps—with long-term care being the most significant—there was little sense of urgency in patching them up because there was every expectation of building on this foundation. Elite conventional wisdom held that Medicare was the first step toward national health insurance for all. The elderly came first because they were most in need, but soon coverage would spread to other groups, eventually becoming universal. In addition to extending health insurance to the non-elderly, it was also anticipated that what holes remained in coverage for seniors would be patched.

This expansionary assumption was predicated on two divergent intellectual foundations. From one perspective, modern societies were seen as progressing in a more-or-less standardized manner. The fact that many European countries (which then, as now, were seen as possessing a certain sophistication and forward-thinking that America lacked) had universal government-financed health systems suggested that it was only a matter of time before the United States—perennially behind the times—caught up and implemented a similar program.[9] The second stream of thought undergirding expectations for Medicare's growth was grounded in the observation—generally made by skeptics of centralized government—that state prerogatives and bureaucracy virtually always grow, frequently with dubious and unintended consequences.[10]

While these two ideas about expansion were rooted in general accounts about the nature of government, they were easy to transpose onto the discussion over Medicare. The program's strongest supporters saw it as merely one small step for the elderly that would be quickly followed by giant leaps for everyone else. Social insurance for seniors was a necessary and politically viable beginning—the low hanging fruit. But the real goal was government-sponsored health insurance for everyone. And in keeping with the idea of progress, many thought such a universal program was not only desirable, but also a natural and inevitable evolutionary outgrowth of a fully developed welfare state.[11]

Similarly, skeptics also saw the 1965 Medicare program as only the beginning. Once instituted, government medicine was destined to follow the slippery slope toward uncontrolled and budget-busting expansion. Political scientist James Q. Wilson, for instance, viewed Medicare in the early 1970s as a classic example of a policy with distributed benefits and distributed costs. Such policies, Wilson argued, could be counted on to expand.

> Policies that both confer benefits on, and spread the costs over, large numbers of persons will tend to become easily institutionalized and to produce increases in benefit levels.... In a democratic society, elected legislators have an incentive to raise the value of widely distributed benefits, especially if those benefits are material. Social Security payments are usually increased in election years ... [and] in time, Medicare benefits may also experience more or less automatic increases.[12]

Wilson concluded that while policies with distributed benefits and costs are initially debated on moral and philosophic terms, "subsequent reviews will be debated, if at all, in terms of economic and political benefits."[13]

Even those who doubted extensive future expansion of Medicare viewed long-term care as a probable addition to the array of publicly sponsored benefits available to all seniors. In a 1965 Ways and Means Committee hearing, Representative Harold Collier (R-IL)—who was concerned that unrestrained expansion was inevitable—asked Wilbur Cohen, assistant secretary at the Department of Health and Human Services, whether "you feel that ... within 4 to 6 years this program, if it were passed, would be expanded to full and complete coverage of all types?" Cohen replied that, in general, he did not think so, but that there was one exception.

> [The Medicare proposal] covers a goodly proportion of the total medical care bill for the aged, with what I would say is one exception.... I think there is still left open for decision how to finance both the construction and the cost of long-term care in skilled nursing

home facilities.... [I]f you passed this particular proposal which has a limited posthospitalization convalescent care, or extended care, it might well be that someone would want to come along later and say this care should be covered for a longer period. But generally speaking I would say with this one exception I don't see a clear-cut basis for expansion.[14]

In short, during and immediately after the 1965 Medicare debates on Capitol Hill, many expected future expansion. This included not only expansion of health insurance to non-elderly groups, but also patching up the remaining holes in coverage for seniors, the most prominent of which was long-term care.

Yet that is not the path Medicare took. Instead, expectations of expansion came face to face with tough economic realities once Medicare's enactment gave way to implementation. The program quickly developed a reputation for economic recklessness. Only a few years after it was implemented, its costs had far exceeded expectations and were growing by more than 40 percent annually. By 1969—just four years after enactment—these overruns led Senator Long, chairman of the Finance Committee, to proclaim Medicare a "runaway program." Because of these budget-busting beginnings, the central concern in Medicare policy rapidly shifted toward restraining the program's costs rather than expanding its benefits.[15]

In this post-1965 context, adding a long-term care benefit to Medicare has generally been seen as a risky, unpredictable, and unaffordable commitment. As a result, Medicare expansion has proven to be halting and limited, and long-term care was never brought into the fold despite three potential openings in the late 1980s and early 1990s.[16]

"THAT LAST FULL MEASURE OF SECURITY"? THE MEDICARE CATASTROPHIC COVERAGE ACT (1988)

In 1988, Congress and President Ronald Reagan initiated a major overhaul of Medicare that came to be known as the Medicare Catastrophic

Coverage Act (MCCA).[17] By the mid-1980s, health care costs had risen to the point that out-of-pocket health expenses for seniors were nearly as much as they had been prior to Medicare's enactment. In response, the central objective of this reform effort was to limit seniors' expenses for "catastrophic care." In contrast with private health insurance plans that cap beneficiaries' annual out-of-pocket costs, Medicare's structure required individuals to pay more as they became sicker. As a result, seniors encumbered with catastrophic costs faced the prospect of being financially crippled. In President Reagan's words:

We all know family, friends, or neighbors who have suffered a devastating illness that has destroyed their financial security. As medical science has given us longer lives, we must face the new challenges to ensure that the elderly have security in their old age. A catastrophic illness can be a short-term condition requiring intensive, acute care services or a lingering illness requiring many years of care.... The single common denominator is financial. It can require personal sacrifices that haunt families for the rest of their lives. I am asking Congress to help give Americans that last full measure of security, to provide a health insurance plan that fights the fear of catastrophic illness.

The president proposed adding a modest new Medicare premium payment that would cover acute (i.e., short-term) care needs and asserted that his plan "also aims to improve protection for the general public and for the long-term care of the elderly."[18]

Among the catastrophic costs seniors encountered, long-term care represented (and continues to represent) the most gaping hole in coverage. For seniors with out-of-pocket expenses exceeding $2,000 annually, long-term care represented more than 80 percent of such costs.[19] Representative Pepper drafted an amendment to include a new long-term care benefit in the MCCA and argued that "it would be a tragedy to accept minor reform at a time when the country is overwhelmingly supportive of meaningful change." Under Pepper's plan, this benefit would have been financed by eliminating the cap on earnings subject to the Medicare payroll tax (in effect, raising taxes on high earners). But the proposal met stiff resistance from the White House and the Democratic congressional leadership, both of which were insisting on a deficit-neutral bill. Eventually, House Speaker Jim Wright (D-TX) persuaded Pepper to drop the amendment by promising him a future vote on a long-term care benefit.[20] Freed of its costly long-term care provision, the MCCA passed easily and established new benefits to combat rising out-of-pocket costs for hospital stays and physician care. A new prescription drug benefit was to be phased in.

The law quickly became a catastrophe in its own right. It was extremely unpopular with elders for two reasons. For many, a law that purported to address catastrophic care for seniors but failed to include coverage for long-term care was farcical. Senator James McClure (R-ID), for instance, said: "This law was misnamed from the beginning. It should not be called Medicare Catastrophic Coverage Act.... The catastrophe that most senior citizens fear the most is ... nursing home care."[21]

The foregoing omission—something that would have benefited a wide swath of seniors—contributed to the other major criticism of the law: that seniors would finance the entire program, and their participation was mandatory. Most of the financing—82 percent—was to come from a new "supplemental premium" imposed progressively on the top 40 percent of senior earners. One quarter of those would pay the maximum tax liability of $800 per person.[22]

If the MCCA had included long-term care services (which would have helped a large segment of beneficiaries), that financing structure may well have been acceptable. But the problem was that most of the seniors on the hook for paying the MCCA's costs would see little if any direct benefit because most of them had supplemental insurance that already offered the new MCCA benefits—62 percent of Medicare enrollees had supplemental private insurance and one-third were covered through an employer or former employer.[23] In effect, then, the MCCA's financing structure meant that those least in need of the new benefits would be paying nearly all of the costs.

Five months after the MCCA passed, "seniors were in open revolt."[24] The pushback reached its peak in a surreal incident featuring the chairman of the Ways and Means Committee, Representative Dan Rostenkowski (D-IL). As he was leaving a meeting in Chicago, an angry contingent of about 200 elders confronted the prominent MCCA supporter. He "was booed and followed down the street by a group of screaming elderly people.... Several dozen people shouted 'Liar!' 'Impeach!' and 'Recall!'" When the congressman got into his car, the protesting senior citizens blocked it, hit it with picket signs, and pounded on the windows. At that point, Rostenkowski got out of the car and attempted to flee on foot. The band of elders followed in hot pursuit until he and his driver reconnected down the street. "The Congressman got back in and the car sped away." In addressing the incident, Rostenkowski told the press: "I don't think [the protesters] understand what's going on. That's too bad."[25] He had a point. While outrage over the MCCA was widespread amongst the elderly, the law actually would have provided about 60 percent of seniors with net benefits.[26]

Be that as it may, the bulk of the MCCA was formally repealed less than a month after the Rostenkowski incident. However, one aspect of the law that managed to survive was funding and authority for a commission—known as the Pepper Commission—to study and make recommendations for health reform that would address long-term care.

It is worth mentioning one noteworthy sideshow in the MCCA debacle. Amidst mounting criticism but prior to its repeal, some MCCA detractors suggested a potential compromise: make the program optional. This proposal was appealing because it would permit those seniors who were upset about being compelled to participate the opportunity to opt out. However, the idea never got off the ground because it would have undermined the program's financing. As noted health policy journalist Julie Rovner explained: "Making the program truly voluntary, as many senior citizens advocated, would have been financially untenable. Only those most likely to need the benefits would opt in, leaving too small a pool over which to spread costs."[27] Due to this obvious problem, the idea of transforming the MCCA into a voluntary program was discarded.

The concept of optional participation, however, was not dead. It would be revived some twenty years later.

A "FLOOR OF PROTECTION" FROM THE "HEALTH-CARE FAIRY": THE PEPPER COMMISSION (1990)

The Pepper Commission—officially known as the U.S. Bipartisan Commission on Comprehensive Health Care—was the result of the MCCA's lone unrepealed provision. The study group was made up of interested members of Congress, and it issued its report in 1990.[28] Long-term care constituted the centerpiece of the commission's work, and the group was unified in concluding "that federal action is essential to change the nation's fundamentally flawed approach to long-term care financing." To meet this challenge the group considered and discarded several possibilities. A "two-tiered system"—with enhanced Medicaid protections for the low-income population and the promotion of private coverage for the better-off—was rejected because it amounted to a mere extension of the status quo and would simply "repeat the nation's unfortunate experience in health care." Likewise, encouraging private savings was rejected because it would focus attention on the "expensive and largely unpredictable" multiyear nursing home stays experienced by "the unlucky few" rather than on spreading risk among the many facing a range of possible limitations. Finally, the commission rejected a comprehensive public insurance program both because it would be costly and because it would offer full financial protection to everyone, including those who could easily afford to pay for private coverage on their own.[29]

Instead, the commission championed a limited social insurance program geared toward meeting the diverse range of long-term care needs. For those requiring home- or community-based care or up to three months of nursing home care, the group recommended a full social insurance program regardless of income. Like Medicare, all but the poorest recipients would be required to contribute to the cost of their care. Those requiring more than three months in a nursing home would have been "guaranteed an ample" means-tested "floor of protection against impoverishment" beginning at $30,000 for individuals or $60,000 for couples (not including their homes, which were also protected). That threshold was relatively generous, approximately equaling the lifetime savings for three-fifths of the elderly population in 1990 and fifteen times today's

Medicaid asset limit. The commission also recommended incentivizing private coverage for those seeking additional protection through revising tax codes, enhancing oversight of insurance companies, and offering consumer counseling.[30]

However, when it came to funding these recommendations, the commission was plagued by bitter infighting and was unable to reach a consensus. As a result, the final report offered only the sketchiest of parameters. While it recognized that substantial new expenditures—estimated at $42.8 billion for 1990—were required, the commission did not specify a funding mechanism. The closest it came was to vaguely recommend that any such mechanism be progressive, draw contributions from people of all ages, and adapt as needed by increasing revenue to cover benefits.[31]

The group's report then abruptly concluded, stating that "Congress called upon the Commission to recommend legislation to ensure all Americans coverage for health and long-term care. With this report, the Commission fulfills its task."[32] Many disagreed. While the Pepper Commission had made specific policy recommendations, its inability to identify and agree on specific funding recommendations for the ambitious new program was widely seen as a failure. Prominent members of Congress—including commission members—declared the report "dead on arrival," and Representative Pete Stark (D-CA) alleged that some of his commission colleagues seemingly believed "in a health-care fairy."[33] No further action was taken, and the commission's report was left to gather dust. But while the Pepper Commission's proposal may have been dead to the 101st Congress, a number of its key themes would be resurrected a few years later for the long-term care component of the Clinton health reform push.

THE CLINTON HEALTH REFORM EFFORT (1993–1994)

There was no guarantee that long-term care would be included in the Clinton health reform proposal. One official involved in crafting the administration's plan argued that "long-term care was not intellectually central to health reform, defined as providing health care to the uninsured and controlling acute-care costs."[34] Others worried about overreaching and that adding long-term care would make the overhaul too costly. However, a long-term care component was ultimately included, largely for political reasons. The administration was anxious to obtain the support of the elderly and their powerful advocacy groups. Long-term care was the price for that support because seniors already had Medicare and would not benefit from the Clinton plan's other provisions.[35]

Because long-term care was something of an afterthought relative to acute care, four fundamental policy questions still needed to be addressed during the health reform process in 1993—issues that continue to stake out the realm of available policy options for long-term care today. First, should the program be exclusively for the elderly or for all people with disabilities? While the Pepper Commission recommended including young disabled persons, most previous long-term care proposals had been geared toward the elderly alone. Second, should the long-term care component provide institutional (e.g., nursing home) or non-institutional services? Third, should the program be based on private insurance, like the proposed acute care reform, or be public? Fourth, should the program be means-tested or universal? To confront these choices and formulate a specific policy proposal, a long-term care workgroup was created and was composed of a few dozen policy experts drawn primarily from the Department of Health and Human Services, think tanks, and various other analysis organizations.

The workgroup proposed a long-term care package with four elements. The centerpiece was the Home and Community-Based Services Program. This component would have provided a non-institutional, non-means-tested, public long-term care program available to disabled individuals of any age. The states would have been tasked with administering the program, but almost all of the financing would have come from Washington. A second element of the package would have established national standards for private long-term care insurance policies and created tax incentives for individuals, employers, and the insurance industry. A third element sought to tweak Medicaid rules governing nursing home care. Finally, the plan offered tax credits for personal assistance services.[36]

Several of the bills reported out of committee included the workgroup's long-term care proposal. But it all became moot when "Hillarycare" collapsed in dramatic fashion without so much as a floor vote in Congress.[37]

IT'S LARGELY ABOUT MONEY: LESSONS FROM FAILED EFFORTS TO CREATE A NATIONAL LONG-TERM CARE PROGRAM

These failures to adopt a national long-term care program carried key political lessons that were internalized by the leading CLASS advocates. CLASS was never viewed as an ideal program from a pure policy perspective. Its chief virtue was its political viability. And the lessons that informed the crafting of a politically viable proposal were learned through the experiences of failing to enact previous long-term care plans. This feature of the CLASS experience carries insights for our general understanding of how learning influences policymaking. Most scholarship on the role of learning in social and health policy is attuned to the feedback effects that existing policy has on future policymaking.[38] To the extent policy failure is encompassed in this work, it is in the context of policies that are successfully implemented but then fail.[39] Because CLASS was shaped by the lessons drawn from previous failures to enact policies, it extends our understanding of the different ways in which learning shapes the policymaking process.

The first and most important of the lessons learned by the advocates who crafted CLASS was that money matters. Though each of the thwarted attempts to create a long-term care program contained their own unique idiosyncrasies, the common impediment was cost. For many on Capitol Hill, the grim realities of cost overruns following Medicare's implementation led to a hasty retreat from bold plans for expansion in favor of a focus on preserving what was already in place by containing costs. This concern over financing was only reinforced by the Pepper Commission and Clinton reform experiences. The Pepper Commission's consensus around its proposed overhaul of long-term care crumbled when attention necessarily shifted toward paying for it. Similarly, the Clinton reform effort reinforced what had by the early 1990s already become painfully obvious: Long-term care is "largely about money."[40] While politically popular in the abstract, the practicalities of addressing it are financially overwhelming.

Worse yet, in the aftermath of the failed Clinton health reform effort, the long-term care component was singled out for blame. The definitive account of that long-term care plan found that because it was so "expensive and add[ed] substantially to the costs of health reform, [it] helped to drag [health reform] down in 1993–94."[41] In the years that followed, that conclusion gained widespread credence in progressive health policy circles.

By the time CLASS was being designed, not only was long-term care perceived to be a costly black hole on its own terms, but many prominent liberals supporting health reform also saw it as a toxic policy area with the potential to drag down another comprehensive health-care bill. In effect, then, over the course of three decades, long-term care had been transformed from a seemingly inevitable addition to Medicare to an untouchable policy area threatening to infect anything it touched. As one aging advocate explained, "There came to be a belief that long-term care doomed the Clinton health reform. It's not true. But [some] thought it was."[42] The advocates realized that this perception—fair or not—could be used as an excuse to exclude long-term care from a future comprehensive reform push. Thus, the aging advocates who designed CLASS were appropriately concerned that whenever the next major attempt at overhauling American health care occurred, they would be pushed aside amidst accusations that they were recklessly holding health reform hostage by insisting that long-term care be included. As a result, they knew that any long-term care proposal would have to be self-financing; it could not require a penny of outside funding.

Following Obama's election and the concomitant preparations for a new health reform push, the fear of being left out proved legitimate. As one CLASS advocate recounted, prominent liberal health reformers were strongly against including long-term care in the Obama legislation: "They said, 'stay out of it.' " The brazen and blunt dismissal of the long-term care community at the beginning of the Obama presidency stung even if it was not unexpected. The aging advocates resented being cast as irresponsible dilettantes willing to blow up the health reform process if their pet interest was not sufficiently catered to. Contrary to that portrayal, the aging advocates behind CLASS saw themselves as unfailingly committed to health reform. But for them, true health reform meant doing something to address one of the largest—albeit largely unrecognized—health challenges facing the country. "We all want health reform," the advocate continued. "The uninsured are number one. But long-term care is also big, and we want something."[43]

These discouraging considerations dovetailed with another lesson dating back to Medicare's inception: Expanding health benefits requires fudging the economic numbers. Had Medicare's true costs been widely known in 1965, it would have never passed. President Lyndon Johnson was fully aware that the program would cost much more than estimated, and he distorted the numbers to get it through Congress. For health policy expert David Blumenthal and political scientist James Morone, this "tension between visionary social reform and economic policy" is the norm when it comes to health reform. As a result, "the most heretical rule in the historical record [is that] expanding health coverage requires presidents who are able and willing to overrule their economic advisors.... [Health reform] never fits the budget, and it never squares with the economic program."[44] This lesson, of course, has applications far beyond the presidency, extending to policy designers and lawmakers as well. It is a lesson the designers of CLASS internalized. As one individual with insider knowledge of CLASS' legislative journey put it: "The Ted Kennedy strategy was to get something on the books and then work it. Once it's there, you can point to it as law and then amend it."[45] More specifically, in the words of one advocate, long-term care's policy history and the widespread skepticism surrounding the issue boiled down to one simple lesson for CLASS: "it couldn't spend a dime."[46]

While addressing the cost concerns that had sunk all previous attempts to enact a national program was the most important lesson the advocates learned, there were other important lessons drawn from long-term care's policy history. One was that mandatory programs are unpopular. The unhappy MCCA experience drove this point home, and it was reinforced with the passage of the Medicare Modernization Act of 2003, which offered a voluntary prescription drug plan within Medicare.[47] This led CLASS advocates to reach a second critical conclusion about their program: "it couldn't have a mandate."[48]

The Clinton reform process carried one other lesson: For long-term care to succeed, it would require a legislative champion. Claude Pepper had filled that role for decades but he had not been replaced. "When he died" in 1989, one health reform participant noted, "we lost our voice. For many years, we sought someone with his commitment, but we never identified a true successor." In 1993–1994, several Democrats were interested in long-term care, but it was not a "make or break" issue for any of them.[49]

The collapse of the MCAA, followed by the failures of the Pepper Commission and the Clinton reform in the span of six years, left many in Washington wary of new efforts to overhaul America's long-term care system. After those failures, legislative action shifted toward modest, incremental tweaks (such as tax incentives for purchasing private long-term care insurance and Medicaid reforms to encourage home and community-based care) that offered more realistic hopes of enactment than did overhauls of the entire system. But while some of these initiatives may have improved care and lowered spending at the margins, they did little to alter the long-term care status quo—a troubling reality defined by relatively few people having long-term care insurance or sufficient savings to cover anticipated needs, with the balance being covered by spiraling Medicaid budgets that threaten to force out other public priorities at the state and national levels.

In sum, to enact meaningful reform, the CLASS advocates realized they needed a work-around solution to avoid the fate of past efforts. Additionally, they needed to address suspicions that long-term care represented a threat that could destroy the entire health reform effort. The key lessons learned by CLASS advocates were that their program "couldn't spend a dime, and it couldn't have a mandate." Any program with any chance of success, they concluded, had to be designed to meet those restrictive—perhaps impossible—constraints. That conclusion dictated CLASS' design.

Learning from Failure

Only Bad Policy Stands a Chance

CLASS was no one's idea of a perfect program. Ideally, the advocates would have preferred a comprehensive, public, non-means-tested social insurance program. Short of that, something like CLASS but with mandated participation would have been far preferable both for maximizing assistance for those with functional limitations and for fiscal solvency (by preventing adverse selection). Yet CLASS' designers felt that a mandate was far too big of a political lift, whereas an optional program would be a much easier sell on Capitol Hill. They also knew their proposal would have to avoid the high price tag and concerns over unpredictability that had thwarted previous attempts to create a national program. Within these significant constraints, the advocates sought to devise a program that could offer meaningful help to people requiring long-term care. The public insurance plan they came up with would be far from the top-to-bottom overhaul they really wanted, but it would be an undeniable step in the right direction.

At the center of the design process behind CLASS was the conviction that political constraints had thwarted prior reform efforts. If CLASS was to succeed where past initiatives had failed, the political prerequisites were to create a program that was optional and that paid for itself. If that meant sacrificing a fiscally sound program for one that might be able to slip its way through Congress, it was a price worth paying. After all, once the

program was on the books, it could be amended or changed administratively. And fixing a law was much easier than passing one.

THE MISSING PIECES: PRESCRIPTION DRUGS
AND LONG-TERM CARE

Organized interests are seen as drivers of policy development—particularly
for expansions of social programs. Interest groups are often able to deci-
sively influence the policy process by lobbying, launching publicity opera-
tions, and donating to political campaigns. In the broadest sense, interest
groups are said to be capable of overwhelming an inattentive public with
intensity and organization, even when pursuing unpopular policies.[1]
Within this interest group orbit, the aging coalition—the "gray lobby"—is
renowned for its political influence, and AARP, formerly the American
Association of Retired Persons, is frequently described as the most powerful of all interest groups.[2]

Following Medicare's enactment, aging groups saw long-term care and
prescription drugs as their two highest priorities. But despite the gray lobby's reputation for power and influence, winning policy victories in these
areas proved difficult. Initial expectations that Medicare would quickly
expand to include more groups as well as these additional benefits fell
victim to the program's cost overruns and the resulting focus on reining
in expenses.

By the time the Clinton health reform effort collapsed in the early 1990s,
the aging organizations—in a triage mentality—consciously decided to
de-emphasize long-term care and focus their efforts on prescription drugs.
The repeated failures to enact a major long-term care program had been
profoundly disappointing and left many concluding that the policy area
simply presented too many political obstacles. In particular, advocates
determined that it was difficult to mobilize public support. They concluded that Americans avoid thinking about long-term care because doing
so requires confronting one's own morbidity and mortality. The policy area
is also difficult because it is inherently expensive and involves tensions

between the private sector and government. As one advocate explained, relative to long-term care, "prescription drugs was easier. People understood it. People who would never complain about long-term care were complaining about prescription drugs."[3] Not only did people understand prescription drugs better, but they also dubiously perceived them to be something that more Medicare beneficiaries needed. That was because a large majority of seniors take at least one prescription medication, while at any one time only a small percentage reside in a nursing home (the most recognizable form of long-term care). Of course, the lifetime likelihood of needing long-term care is also very high and is quite likely to be far more costly. But people don't calculate or acknowledge those cumulative likelihoods and costs. A final consideration—and another contrast with long-term care—was that, because most health insurance plans offered prescription coverage, it seemed only natural and consistent for Medicare to have a parallel offering. Zeroing in on prescription drugs eventually proved successful when, with AARP support, President George W. Bush signed the Medicare Modernization Act of 2003 to create Part D of Medicare.

With that, long-term care was left as the last remaining top-tier risk for elders. However, the old roadblocks remained.

THE FRIDAY GROUP: AN UNLIKELY ALLIANCE

In the post-Medicare Part D era, the aging advocates who would go on to be part of the CLASS effort knew several things. As noted, the lessons they'd drawn from long-term care's policy history established some basic requirements for any forthcoming policy proposal: no mandatory participation and no price tag. Equally important, they had also learned that they needed a legislative vehicle to move any long-term care proposal. As one advocate emphasized, "post-Clinton, we realized we have to be opportunistic." They concluded that "long-term care wasn't strong enough to go on its own, so we had to piggyback on health care."[4]

These lessons framed the strategic approach to designing CLASS in two important ways. First, there was a realization that the CLASS

Act—whether as a stand-alone bill or having "piggybacked" onto a larger bill—would eventually be scrutinized by the Congressional Budget Office (CBO) and that that agency's report would be absolutely critical to CLASS' political viability. Piggybacking would require that CLASS offer something appealing—namely, savings—that would improve the prospects of passing the larger legislative package. To say the least, generating savings would be a tall task because long-term care had a well-earned reputation for being costly. According to conventional wisdom in Washington, adding a long-term care program offered no upside but carried the disastrous potential to sink a comprehensive health reform package. CLASS' designers had to upend that solidly ingrained perception. To that end, CLASS was crafted with CBO scoring in mind. And because the CBO uses a standard ten-year window to evaluate programs, its scoring system can be gamed quite easily. For policy designers, the key is to fashion a program that is solvent for ten years. Whatever happens in year eleven and thereafter is immaterial insofar as a program's CBO score is concerned. This means that even if economic calamity is a certainty beginning in year eleven, it will not be factored into the all-important score the CBO produces.

Second, the lessons learned from past failures suggested that an alliance between the groups advocating on behalf of the aging and those advocating for the disabled might be mutually beneficial. This notion was counterintuitive because the groups had traditionally had an antagonistic relationship that one advocate characterized as "fighting over Medicaid pennies."[5] The disability advocates tended to view their aging counterparts with envy. From their perspective, the large, politically active membership behind AARP and the other aging organizations translated into unmatchable power, political clout, and appropriations. Additionally, young disabled persons feared being stuck in institutions with old people, which led many disabled groups to identify nursing homes as an enemy. Aging groups, on the other hand, viewed the disability groups dismissively. One advocate explained that the aging groups "saw the disabled community as not like us ... disruptive and [dealing with] mental issues and addiction issues" that were not a concern for the generationally distinct aging population.[6] Yet despite this antagonistic relationship, CLASS offered something compelling to each constituency. For the disabled community, the partnership ensured that the aging lobby's political clout would be directed in a way that helped rather than hindered their priorities. And for the aging community, the partnership provided the outlines of a legislative vehicle as well as a formidable champion in Senator Ted Kennedy.

Around the time the Medicare Modernization Act was making its way through Congress in 2003, the disability groups—led by organizations such as Arc, United Cerebral Palsy, and Easter Seals—and their allies on Capitol Hill were in the early stages of developing the program that eventually became CLASS.

The driving force behind CLASS from beginning to end was Connie Garner, an indefatigable member of Senator Kennedy's staff and a passionate advocate for the disabled community. In seventeen years on Capitol Hill, she had shepherded numerous high-profile bills into law and presided over the reauthorization of others. Beyond her policy achievements with Kennedy, Garner also had experience at the Department of Education working on issues for disabled children. In addition, she was a practicing nurse and mother to seven kids, including one with a disability. Garner was initially inspired to build on the Americans with Disabilities Act of 1990 and the Kennedy-sponsored (and Garner-spearheaded) Ticket to Work and Work Incentives Improvement Act of 1999, a law designed to allow disabled individuals to be employed without losing Medicaid coverage. Garner's idea for a next step was to target these same people—working-age individuals with disabilities—by establishing a program that would offer a modest daily cash benefit that could be used to cover a wide variety of expenses associated with daily needs.

While Garner and Kennedy originally envisioned a program for disabled individuals in their working years (as opposed to those sixty-five and older), their basic idea also held considerable appeal for the aging groups. Most importantly, the daily cash benefit would provide significant help for elders who needed assistance with some activities of daily living but were still able to live at home (a setting with much lower costs than nursing facilities). Recognizing a mutual interest, the aging groups—most notably AARP and LeadingAge (formerly known as the American Association of

Homes and Services for the Aging)—joined forces with Garner and the disability groups to craft what became the CLASS Act.

For more than two years, the "Friday Group," consisting of Garner and about fifteen representatives of the various organizations, met weekly in Kennedy's Senate office to develop CLASS. This core group of advocates had long experience in the trenches of Washington policymaking, though they eventually stitched together a much broader and more diverse grass-roots coalition of 275 organizations that publicly endorsed the program.

But old habits die hard, and the CLASS alliance was far from seamless. For instance, the aging and disability communities were frequently in conflict concerning revisions to the program's language. The roots of the tension between the two cohorts can be better comprehended by understanding the sometimes imprecise terminology used to describe the overlapping areas of long-term care policy and disability policy. CLASS came to be known as a long-term care program, but it was originally conceived of as a disability program. While the two frames aren't incompatible, they frequently carry different implications. "Long-term care" has traditionally been most closely associated with seniors, even though about one-third of those requiring assistance with activities of daily living are under the age of sixty-five.[7] Policy experts usually have a broader understanding of the term that recognizes those non-senior individuals with disabilities, but to the extent a popular image of long-term care exists, it tends to be centered on nursing homes and the senior citizens who constitute the substantial majority of individuals requiring assistance with activities of daily living. "Disabled," by contrast, has often been used to refer to non-elderly individuals, even though many elderly are, in fact, disabled. Sometimes the distinction is clarified by prefacing "disabled" with "young" or "working." Additionally, while important similarities are found between seniors and non-seniors who need assistance with basic daily activities, there are also key differences. Seniors, for instance, are by definition beyond their normal working years, while many younger individuals with disabilities want to contribute to society and help support themselves and their families by working. Thus, there are certain reasons why the long-term care and disability policy arenas are sometimes considered one in the same, but there are also crucial differences that push against a simple blending of the two. These differences historically pitted the groups against one another and left a legacy of mistrust and resentment that the CLASS alliance diluted but could not entirely overcome.

Yet despite ongoing tensions, the unification held, and the bond between the previously oppositional groups helped CLASS to proceed. Moreover, the partnership managed to create a sense of strength in numbers in the face of a litany of other interests involved in the health policy world that were either ambivalent or hostile to CLASS.

THE NUTS AND BOLTS OF THE CLASS ACT

Though proposals for a "public option" for health insurance were dropped from the Affordable Care Act, the CLASS Act was grounded in that very idea.[8] It was designed to be an optional, publicly administered long-term care insurance program that would be available alongside current offerings in the private market. But there was an important difference between the "public option" proposal for health insurance and the optional CLASS Act. The public option for health insurance would have worked within a marketplace in which everyone was *required* to purchase health insurance through the Affordable Care Act's individual mandate.[9] The "option" would have been to purchase the government's plan or a private plan. With CLASS, on the other hand, there would have been an additional option: nothing. A related difference was consumer demand. Health insurance (even without an individual mandate) is widely desired; most people want it. Comparatively, long-term care insurance could scarcely be more different. While a strong case can be made that people *should* desire it, the reality is that most people don't, be it out of ignorance, confusion, the dysfunctional private market, or some combination of these factors. Thus, the fact that CLASS was designed to be a voluntary program clearly presented adverse selection concerns that were impossible to miss for anyone with knowledge of long-term care or insurance markets. But, as the advocates knew all too well, it was also undeniably true that any proposal that forced people to purchase long-term care insurance (i.e., an individual mandate) would not even receive the dignity of being voted down in Congress; it would simply be ignored. Although a mandatory program was the only financially viable route, an optional program was the only politically viable route.

When CLASS was officially rolled out as a standalone bill (years prior to being attached to the Obama health reform legislation), Senator Kennedy announced: "The bill we propose is a long overdue effort to offer greater dignity, greater hope, and greater opportunity. It makes a simple pact with all Americans – 'If you work hard and contribute, society will take care of you when you fall on hard times.'" In addition, Kennedy said: "The concept is clear, everyone can contribute and everyone can win. We all benefit when no one is left behind." A press release also quoted the sponsor of CLASS in the House, Representative Frank Pallone (D-NJ), as saying, "[a]s America continues to age, we are faced with an impending crisis in long-term care. Today, we offer a new approach that builds upon our existing safety net system and helps our elderly and disabled finance the long-term care they need."[10]

In terms of policy, the idea behind CLASS was to provide a realistic long-term care option for individuals and families lacking the resources to self-finance their care but who were not Medicaid eligible. Under CLASS, any "working" American—defined as someone earning $1,120 annually in any three of the previous five years—age eighteen and over would be eligible to enroll. Beyond that stipulation, there was to be no underwriting. This lack of underwriting was a top priority for the disability groups whose clientele were commonly denied private coverage or faced exorbitant premiums.

The premiums under CLASS, by contrast, would be low—only $30 a month and transmitted through payroll withholding. (Later versions of the program contained higher premiums because it had become clear that the $30 figure was implausible.) For full-time students under twenty-two and those with incomes at or below the poverty line, monthly premiums would be just $5.

CLASS was to be self-sustaining, relying entirely on these premiums to cover its expenses. This design feature sought to allay the worries about costs that had hung over long-term care reform proposals since the Medicare debate in 1965. Yet, with no requirement to enroll, it was never clear how CLASS would be self-sustaining. It was nonetheless routinely presented in this way.

After a five-year "vesting period" of paying into the program (a particularly important feature of CLASS), enrollees who were disabled and struggling with two or more activities of daily living would receive a daily cash benefit of either $50 or $100, based on level of impairment, for the rest of their lives to help fund the services they required. While premiums would be locked in upon enrollment, the daily benefit would be indexed for inflation.[11] This policy design meant that some participants who paid as little as $300 in premiums over five years could thereafter receive $18,250 to $36,500 annually until death.

Despite these provisions that would suggest a costly program requiring significant government subsidies, CLASS managed to avoid the appearance of being a fiscal liability. The key to this improved image relative to earlier long-term care proposals was the five-year waiting period before enrollees would become eligible for benefits. Waiting periods are common enough in the private long-term care insurance market, as they are in other areas such as pension plans. Even Social Security had an initial three-year pre-funding period when it was first implemented. So conceptually there was nothing atypical here. But, as previously noted, private long-term care insurance plans have waiting periods of days, not years. Indeed, it is rare for a private plan to require a vesting period in excess of 100 days. Thus, the five-year vesting period for CLASS was quite unusual in the context of long-term care insurance, yet it was a critical feature of the program's design and the key to its professed "savings."

Members of the Friday Group were well aware that the CBO uses a ten-year window to evaluate the budgetary implications of proposed programs. Including a five-year vesting period in CLASS meant that for the first half of that scoring window, the program would be stockpiling premium payments without having to issue any benefits. While benefit payments would begin in year six, it was anticipated that those stockpiled funds would not be depleted until the CBO's ten-year window had closed. As such, CLASS was expected to register savings when the CBO evaluated it and reported on its ten-year budgetary outlook. Of course, such an evaluation would obscure the program's true costs following the first five years. But on its face, the CBO would report savings. And it would be that hard number produced by the CBO—not any caveats the agency explained in the fine print—that would be critical for CLASS' political viability. Therefore, the Friday Group was optimistic that CLASS would not only avoid the grim fiscal implications that had dragged down earlier long-term care proposals, but also that it would appear to generate savings—potentially big savings—when it went through the CBO scoring process.

FROM KENNEDY'S OFFICE TO THE SENATE FLOOR

CLASS was first introduced in Congress in 2005 by Senators Ted Kennedy and Mike DeWine (R-OH), though it went nowhere.[12] Two years later, Kennedy reintroduced the bill in the Senate, and a House version was offered by Representative Pallone.[13] In his reintroduction, Kennedy reiterated that the typical monthly premium would be $30 and the daily benefits would be $50 or $100 depending on level of need. At this time, CLASS was primarily touted as a bill for the "working disabled." In a 2007 speech on the Senate floor, for instance, Kennedy described the program's benefits for this group while making no reference to the aging community. CLASS, he said, "builds on the promise and possibilities of the Americans with Disabilities Act.... Too often [people] have to give up the American Dream, the dignity of a job, a home, and a family, so they can qualify for Medicaid." Continuing, Kennedy noted that CLASS "will strengthen job opportunities for people with disabilities.... They have so much to contribute and the bill will help them do it." Kennedy's only explicit mention of "long-term care" came in the context of working-age individuals: "[CLASS] will save on the mushrooming health care costs for Medicaid, the Nation's primary insurer of long-term care services, which also forces beneficiaries to give up their jobs and live in poverty before they become eligible for assistance."[14] Kennedy's initial rhetorical focus on disability rather than aging is not surprising because the program's basic concept was originally formulated by disability advocates and because Kennedy himself had a long history of engagement with disability issues.

In the years that followed, the language surrounding CLASS became less explicitly focused on the "working disabled." Gradually, the more generic rhetoric of "long-term care" became the norm. For instance, in a typical formulation, Senator Paul Kirk (D-MA, Kennedy's temporary replacement in 2009) opened a floor debate about CLASS as follows:

> [A]pproximately 200 million of our citizens are elderly or disabled. These are not mere statistics. They are family members and loved ones—vulnerable, challenged, and often forgotten. But they were not forgotten by their friend and advocate, Senator Ted Kennedy.... Sadly, millions of seniors and persons living with disabilities struggle to obtain the services and supports they need to live fulfilling lives and to remain in their communities among their friends and families—in what they hoped would be their productive golden years.... Aging baby boomers and longer lifespans will increase the demand for long-term care dramatically for decades to come.... The CLASS Act is designed specifically to remedy this looming crisis by giving people an affordable option other than Medicaid.[15]

This revised rhetorical framework carried the advantage of appealing to the aging groups that, for obvious reasons, are not oriented toward the needs of those in their prime working years. Moreover, it highlighted the unlikely alliance between the previously antagonistic groups.

That alliance had endured against long odds to see a vague idea hashed out in Kennedy's office get introduced as formal legislation. But as a stand-alone bill in the 109th (2005–2006) and 110th (2007–2008) Congresses,

CLASS had generated no momentum and had no realistic prospect of advancing. The advocates recognized that CLASS was too low salience to move through Congress on its own. Finding a home for the program in another piece of legislation was clearly the only hope. During the 2008 presidential campaign, an obvious prospect emerged.

CLASS on Capitol Hill, Part 1

*Dodging Committee Jurisdiction
and the Number Crunchers*

In 2008, the major Democratic presidential candidates had made comprehensive health reform a centerpiece of their campaigns, and by the time
Barack Obama took the oath of office in 2009, it was clear that it would
be the centerpiece of his legislative agenda. The advocates who designed
CLASS recognized this was the vehicle they'd been waiting for to carry
their program across the finish line. They also had reason to believe that
this time would be different from the previous attempts to overhaul long-
term care. That's because CLASS, once it went through the CBO scoring
process, was likely to have something valuable to offer, namely, projected
savings that could be used to help pay for health reform.

The 2009–2010 national health reform effort coalesced around three
pieces of legislation forged in congressional committees holding jurisdiction over health care. In the Senate, separate processes played out in
the Finance Committee and the Health, Education, Labor, and Pensions
(HELP) Committee. The three relevant House committees—Energy and
Commerce, Ways and Means, and Education and Labor—acted more col-
laboratively. Each drafted language dealing with the issues in their jurisdiction and then combined them into a single bill.

For all the focus on health reform, few in Washington's political and policy circles were eager to see long-term care included in the discussion. The

top priority for the White House and Democrats in Congress was securing health insurance for as many of the estimated fifty million people lacking it as possible. Many recognized that long-term care was a serious issue, but they thought it should be addressed separately from health reform. It was also easy to ignore because it generated little public outcry, and there were no easy or obvious ways to solve what was widely regarded as an intractable problem. Additionally, as previously discussed, some blamed long-term care for thwarting the Clinton initiative and worried that including it as part of the new health reform effort carried high risks and low rewards. Those outside the long-term care orbit generally felt that if the issue was to be addressed at all, it should wait until after comprehensive health reform was completed lest it complicate that more important objective.

For many who played a role in passing the Affordable Care Act, the inclusion of CLASS remains a source of frustration and is cited as one reason why the Affordable Care Act has struggled to garner legitimacy and public support. As one congressional staffer who was closely involved in developing the Affordable Care Act said: "[CLASS] wasn't thought through.... It was globbed on. It didn't belong in health reform."[1] Nonetheless, this advocate-designed, long-shot policy idea with scant congressional support in general—and even less in the context of the 2009–2010 health reform process—made it all the way to the Affordable Care Act's East Room signing ceremony.

SHELL GAME: CLASS IN THE HOUSE

CLASS' House sponsor, Representative Frank Pallone, was well positioned to champion the program from his seat on the Energy and Commerce Committee. Committee chair Henry Waxman (D-CA)—a Pepper Commission veteran—was supportive, and member John Dingell (D-MI), another influential legislator with an interest in long-term care, was a key partner. These leading figures on Energy and Commerce thought that without CLASS, long-term care would be unjustly left out of health reform entirely.

CLASS supporters on Energy and Commerce, however, were boxed in by their committee colleagues and by committee jurisdiction. Other committee members—particularly the sizable "Blue Dog" contingent of fiscally conservative Democrats—were seen as roadblocks likely to take issue with the program's financing scheme. And even with attention focused on the larger issues surrounding health reform, CLASS supporters thought slipping the Pallone bill through Energy and Commerce would be difficult or impossible. Committee jurisdiction also constrained CLASS backers because all legislation with revenue implications had to pass through the Ways and Means Committee. It was for this reason that CLASS had previously been referred to both committees the two times Pallone had introduced it as a stand-alone measure. This meant that Energy and Commerce could not unilaterally move Pallone's original version of CLASS along. And that presented a problem because the Ways and Means Committee, chaired by Charles Rangel (D-NY), was, at best, unenthusiastic about CLASS. For years, Rangel had advocated a single-payer health plan that included long-term care coverage. To Rangel, ex-Pepper Commission member Pete Stark, and other prominent Ways and Means Democrats, CLASS paled next to the old dream of a social insurance model for long-term care or a program with mandatory participation.[2]

According to several Democratic staffers with direct knowledge of the House process, this meant that Energy and Commerce "had to restructure CLASS for getting it in around Ways and Means."[3] To pull off this avoidance of Rangel's committee and to avoid the ire of their own Blue Dogs, CLASS supporters in Energy and Commerce drafted what they called a "shell" of the CLASS program that lacked any financing provisions or wording about how to pay for the program, thereby sidestepping any revenue implications that would cause it to fall within the purview of Ways and Means. The CLASS shell passed through Energy and Commerce on a voice vote. The program's supporters thought they would have also prevailed on a roll call vote for the shell, though not for the full-fledged CLASS Act (including the financing provisions).

When the House committees combined their various provisions into a single health reform bill for the full chamber, the CLASS shell was included due to jurisdictional privilege. The carefully crafted shell, because it was written to be fully within Energy and Commerce jurisdiction, gave Pallone, Dingell, and Waxman "a leg up" in arguing for its inclusion in the combined House bill.[4] Ultimately, then, the House's version of health reform—the Affordable Health Care for America Act—included a CLASS provision devised by Energy and Commerce that was "totally open ended . . . to avoid Ways and Means."[5] As another staffer explained: "Frank Pallone had to advocate strongly to get the shell through—not the [full] CLASS Act. It was an uphill battle to get [the shell] through Energy and Commerce. . . . That's all we could do. We couldn't go into Ways and Means jurisdiction, and we couldn't get [the full version of] CLASS through [the Energy and Commerce] Committee."[6]

This outcome in the House marked a big victory for CLASS supporters. Theoretically, CLASS did not have to be in the House legislation so long as it made it into the Senate bill, and, in that regard, it was anticipated that the full-fledged version of CLASS would be included in the Kennedy-chaired HELP Committee legislation. Yet CLASS supporters still felt it was important to get some version of the program into the House package in preparation for the expected conference committee which would mold the separate House- and Senate-passed bills into a final, single piece of legislation to be sent to the president for his signature. If the House legislation lacked any long-term care language, CLASS' status might be questioned by opponents, who would argue that the House had purposefully chosen not to address long-term care and that CLASS was therefore inappropriate for consideration in the conference committee—assuming health reform got that far.[7] The shell more than met this low threshold. The lack of financing details was not considered important at this time because, as one congressional staffer explained, "there was every expectation of a conference committee. So [the plan was to] just get something through and deal with it then."[8] Assuming HELP did its job on the Senate side, all the details intentionally left out of the Energy and Commerce shell would reappear in the conference committee.

EVADING FISCAL OVERSIGHT IN THE SENATE

CLASS endured a more grueling process in the Senate. As in the House, committee jurisdiction was a defining feature of the program's path through the upper chamber. Two Senate committees have sometimes overlapping jurisdiction over health issues. The Finance Committee oversees health programs paid for through taxes or trust funds, while HELP's jurisdiction includes health, aging, and disability measures.

Yet while both committees claim jurisdiction over health issues, a program like CLASS would typically have to pass muster with Finance. That is because the monthly premiums for individuals enrolled in CLASS were to be paid for by payroll deductions, which falls squarely on Finance Committee turf. The previous three times the CLASS Act was introduced as a stand-alone bill (in 2005, 2007, and 2009) it was referred exclusively to Finance (as was a 2011 bill to repeal the program). Further illustrating that CLASS clearly fell within the jurisdiction of Finance, in a 2007 HELP Committee hearing on the program, Senator Tom Harkin (D-IA) repeatedly emphasized to the advocates that "we really need you to press forward on getting the Finance Committee of the Senate to have hearings" on CLASS.[9] As one congressional staffer put it: "The idea of a program with payroll withholding to not be with Finance is offensive."[10]

However, Finance and its chair, Max Baucus (D-MT), were opposed to CLASS, which meant that the program would go nowhere on the conventional path through the committee system. But fortunately for CLASS, its biggest champion was the HELP Committee chair. Additionally, as one congressional staffer emphasized, "[i]t's not a random set of Senators on HELP. The [HELP] Democrats are traditionally more progressive and more open to Ted Kennedy's agenda" than the rest of the Democratic caucus.[11] With Majority Leader Harry Reid's approval, Kennedy was permitted to carry CLASS exclusively through the HELP committee during the 2009–2010 health reform process. Avoiding Finance was important for CLASS, but it was also highly unusual, and that fact, at least for some, stirred tensions between the committees. One Hill staffer with close knowledge of the process on the Senate side saw the exclusion of Finance as "laughable" as well as a blatant evasion of the committee tasked with ensuring that proposed programs are fiscally sound.[12]

As HELP chair, Kennedy was in a position to ensure that CLASS was included in the initial June 2009 draft of the committee's health reform bill. Kennedy's influence also allowed him to assemble a staff that was committed to the program. The linchpin was Connie Garner, who drafted the CLASS Act and shepherded it through the lawmaking process. With the possible exception of her boss, she played the most pivotal role in taking the long-shot bill drawn up by the Friday Group all the way to President Obama's desk.

Yet Kennedy and Garner could carry CLASS only so far. Just because the program was included in the initial HELP health reform package did not mean that it would make it out of the committee, let alone be part of the final Senate bill that combined the best elements that emerged from the separate processes playing out in Finance and HELP. Then, in June, at the height of the committee deliberations, CLASS' legislative champion was permanently sidelined. Though his spirit would be invoked throughout the final months of the health reform process, Kennedy's battle against brain cancer necessitated a move home to his family's Hyannis Port compound. Within the HELP Committee, his longtime friend and ally Chris Dodd (D-CT) became acting chair and CLASS' chief proponent in the Senate.[13]

A "DEATH SPIRAL"? THE FIRST RED FLAGS

As the health reform process dominated Washington in the late spring and early summer of 2009, two actuarial assessments laid bare the economic problems of CLASS and threatened to undermine the program's momentum. These assessments, and several others that came later, were critical features in the lawmaking process behind both CLASS and the Affordable Care Act as a whole, and they played a central role in debates on Capitol Hill and in efforts by both the bill's supporters and opponents to harness public opinion. While much of this actuarial back-and-forth over CLASS took place out of the public eye, the various reports pointed toward serious financing difficulties and damaged the program's credibility in Congress. As a potential addition to the final legislative package, CLASS' economic viability (or lack thereof) also carried budgetary implications for the health reform process as a whole.

The first warning came in May 2009 from Richard Foster, the chief actuary at the Centers for Medicare and Medicaid Services (an agency within the Department of Health and Human Services). In an internal email to colleagues, he reported that his preliminary finding was that it "may be impossible" for CLASS to be actuarially self-sustaining because it was likely to attract only enrollees who already qualified for benefits. Foster asserted that "this could be a terminal problem for this proposal." Additionally, he pointed to CLASS' requirement that enrollees pay into the system for five years prior to receiving benefits. From an actuarial standpoint, this provision was important because, as previously discussed, it meant the program would be collecting premiums for five years without paying any benefits. That vesting period would distort the attempt by the Congressional Budget Office (CBO) to forecast CLASS' future sustainability and its true costs due to the agency's standard ten-year scoring window for evaluating such programs. Foster suggested that without required participation, not enough people would sign up for CLASS and that all the resources built up during the program's initial five years would quickly be depleted, possibly within the first several months of CLASS' sixth year when benefit checks would start being issued. An "insurance death spiral" would result. Foster then described a best case scenario in which CLASS attracted broad enrollment:

[S]uppose that a significant number of people without any limitations in [activities of daily living] could be persuaded to participate in the program. How many people would be needed to cover the benefit costs for those qualifying as beneficiaries? For the sake of illustration, suppose 10 million people qualify for benefits of $50 per day (annual cost of $182.5 billion). About 234 million people, paying premiums of $65 per month, would be needed to cover this cost (ignoring administrative expenses). The size of the U.S. population aged 20 and over is about 225 million, and about 165 million of these are employed. This rough—but probably not unrealistic—example further calls into question the feasibility of the maximum financing versus the minimum benefits.

It amounted to a devastating assessment from the key shop within the Obama administration's Department of Health and Human Services. At this point, though, Foster's concerns were not known outside of the Centers for Medicare and Medicaid Services, and he was careful to note that his "quick read" may have overlooked important details.[14]

Several weeks later in early July, the CBO weighed in for the first time with a formal assessment that at first glance appeared to be far more positive, but that was actually fairly consistent with that of Foster. Throughout the health reform process, assessments from the CBO were particularly important because of the agency's reputation for producing apolitical, legitimate, and trustworthy analysis. The CBO officially scored CLASS as providing $58 billion in savings over its first ten years.[15] However, the CBO—like Foster—also noted that the estimated reduction in the ten-year budget window was due to the five-year vesting requirement that distorted the program's true costs. The CBO concluded that "if the Secretary did not modify the program to ensure its actuarial soundness, it would add to future federal budget deficits in a large and growing fashion beginning a few years beyond the 10-year budget window." And even if the secretary did make changes to address the program's solvency, CLASS "might—or might not—add to future budget deficits."[16]

In short, these reports from Foster and the CBO indicated that the central problem for CLASS was that its design would lead to debilitating adverse selection that would render it economically unworkable. Because participation in CLASS was optional, those with long-term care needs would be much more likely to enroll. To cover the costs of providing benefits for this disproportionately needy group of enrollees, premiums would have to be raised. Higher premiums would, in turn, discourage healthy people from signing up or maintaining their coverage, thereby spurring a vicious cycle in which premiums skyrocketed and enrollment of healthy, non-benefit-eligible individuals plummeted. Both Foster and the CBO predicted this calamity; the only difference between them was whether the program would collapse immediately upon initiating benefit payments in year six or manage to limp along in the black for a few years beyond the CBO's ten-year scoring window.

Despite these gloomy assessments of CLASS' long-term viability, the program's supporters celebrated the CBO report. After all, on its face, the CBO reported that CLASS would save $58 billion. That figure was—as one official from the Centers for Medicare and Medicaid Services wrote in an email at the time—the "bottom line."[17]

And the good news kept coming. Immediately after the CBO unveiled its projection of CLASS' $58 billion in savings over ten years, the White House officially came out in support of the program and having it added to the health reform legislation.[18]

"CLASS ACT—BAIT AND SWITCH?" THE HELP MARKUP AND JUDD GREGG'S AMENDMENT NO. 6

One day after the CBO released its initial assessment, the markup began for the HELP Committee's bill. The key moment for CLASS came during a fifty-minute exchange on July 7, 2009. Taking issue with the reported savings and obscured long-range costs generated by the CBO's ten-year projection, Senator Judd Gregg (R-NH) offered Amendment No. 6, which proposed replacing the bill's language that identified the then-current estimate of monthly premiums averaging $65 with a directive that the Health and Human Services Secretary set premiums in a manner that ensured the program would be solvent for seventy-five years. Pointing to a bar chart titled "CLASS Act – Bait and Switch?" Gregg argued:

> Yes, in the first ten years this thing makes money. But over [40] years, it's a $2 trillion unfunded liability. . . . Now, the Chairman makes the comment: "Well, we have language in here that the Secretary must

adjust and make it solvent." Well, why would you start off with a program that's insolvent and then tell the Secretary, "Oh, you've got to adjust for solvency"? Let's start up front with solvency. . . . There seems to be a consistency of thought around here that we should have a solvent program. I'm not opposing the program. I'm just saying let's have a solvent program.[19]

The amendment was intensely debated for more than thirty minutes. Gregg—prominently joined by Senator Tom Coburn (R-OK)—argued that "from day one you know this program is insolvent . . . once you get outside the ten-year window." They contended that the revised $65 premium (up from the original $30) was a "charade" and that ten-year forecasts of CLASS savings were "absurd on their face" given the five-year vesting period's distorting effects. It amounted to knowingly creating an insolvent program that would require a federal bailout to the tune of trillions of dollars. Gregg argued that the only honest way to score the program was to employ a seventy-five-year scoring window rather than the ten-year CBO standard. The longer timeframe, he maintained, made more sense because it accounted both for people paying in and for people collecting benefits.[20]

Sensing that CLASS was on the verge of being lost, the acting committee chair, Senator Dodd, with Connie Garner's approval, asked Gregg whether he would support CLASS if his amendment was adopted. Gregg replied that he would. Leaping at the opportunity to keep the program alive, Dodd promptly called for a voice vote in which Amendment No. 6 passed.[21]

This meant that CLASS' place in the HELP bill had been secured. But it came at a high price. The seventy-five-year solvency requirement inserted a new standard that, if left in place, would not be easy to meet for those tasked with implementing the program. Some CLASS supporters were immediately concerned. "We saw [the solvency requirement] as a problem right away," recounted one advocate, "but we thought it would get stripped in conference [committee]. But it let [CLASS] move forward" when it otherwise might have been killed during the HELP markup.[22]

Gregg's Amendment No. 6 has been an ongoing source of controversy and is among the more intriguing subplots within the Affordable Care Act's lawmaking process. Accounts differ sharply on whether Gregg was duped into setting the stage for CLASS' inclusion in the health reform law or whether he cleverly inserted language destined to sabotage a flawed program. The bumbling Gregg version posits that CLASS was on the verge of being stripped from the HELP bill when he offered his amendment. Gregg assumed the amendment had no chance of being accepted and offered it merely as a way to pile on and highlight CLASS' economic fallacies. However, the tables were turned when Dodd surprised Gregg by accepting the amendment. Furious Republican staffers recognized what was going on before Gregg did but they had to helplessly watch in horror as the New Hampshire senator steered the plane into the mountain. Had he not agreed to support CLASS in exchange for the inclusion of his amendment, the program might well have died right there in the HELP Committee room. Gregg's political ineptness may have been the only thing that could have saved the program he was trying to kill.[23] And, nearly as damning, his amendment allowed CLASS supporters to begin claiming that the program had bipartisan support and that Gregg had played a key role in designing it. As one advocate recounted, "we hung our hat on that ever after."[24]

Others with knowledge of the markup tell a different story: CLASS was destined to move forward given the widespread sentimental support for granting a dying Kennedy his last wish. Given this unfortunate reality, they explain, Gregg shrewdly introduced an actuarially sound amendment requiring that CLASS either achieve solvency—something that was plainly impossible—or be discarded. Having masterfully maneuvered Dodd into a corner, Gregg forced the Democrats to support what appeared to be a harmless call for fiscal pragmatism that was above reproach. Yet the New Hampshire senator had adroitly planted the seed that would eventually bring down CLASS.[25]

Both versions of the story contain elements of truth. With the possible exception of Gregg himself,[26] no one denies that he was surprised when Dodd agreed to accept his amendment. In adopting the amendment in exchange for Gregg's support of the program, CLASS backers received a political gift enabling them to argue—as they would at every opportunity in the months to follow—that Republicans had helped design CLASS and even suggested a key improvement to fix the program's financing. But even though Amendment No. 6 produced a political dividend for CLASS supporters, it also cast new light on the program's structural problems. The standard ten-year scoring window employed by the CBO was no longer the only frame for viewing CLASS. Gregg's amendment highlighted assertions that if CLASS was examined outside of its first decade, it was clearly a looming financial disaster. More importantly, the amendment established a stringent new standard that would have to be met during implementation unless, as expected, the provision was eliminated during the conference committee.

MORE RED FLAGS—AND EVEN MORE
CBO-CERTIFIED SAVINGS

Just two days after CLASS survived the HELP markup, the behind-the-scenes actuarial assessment dispute ramped up again. Following Foster's initial warnings, the HELP committee had sent two actuarial reports to him and his colleagues at the Centers for Medicare and Medicaid Services that purportedly demonstrated CLASS' viability. The first, a 2008 AARP study, found that the initial version of CLASS (containing a $30 average premium) could work with sufficient enrollment and flexibility with the premium. Nonetheless, the study's modeling showed that "the combination of voluntary enrollment, the prohibition of underwriting, and community rating will eventually lead to a deterioration of the pool of enrollees and an unsustainable situation with respect to the premium. Options for curing this problem include more significant governmental subsidies . . . or making the program mandatory."[27] The other report HELP forwarded to Foster was conducted by the Moran Company and predicted (based on, as will be seen, inapplicable assumptions) that a program like CLASS would be solvent and would cut Medicaid's long-term care expenditures in half.[28]

After examining these HELP-provided AARP and Moran studies, Foster remained unconvinced. In another internal email on July 9 that was shared with officials at the Department of Health and Human Services and the HELP Committee, he reported that despite having reviewed the studies, he was still "very doubtful that [CLASS] is sustainable." Foster concluded that the AARP and Moran studies were irrelevant insofar as they were being used to suggest that CLASS was viable. Foster explained that the new studies were beside the point because they were predicated on unrealistic enrollment figures. AARP ran its numbers based on 40–100 percent enrollment, while Moran assumed that enrollment would be mandatory.[29] By contrast, no one thought CLASS would get anywhere close to 40 percent enrollment, let alone 100 percent; something between 2 and 5 percent seemed more realistic, even according to CLASS' proponents.[30] Foster ominously concluded: "Thirty-six years of actuarial experience lead me to believe that [CLASS] would collapse in short order and require significant Federal subsidies to continue."[31]

In the midst of this pushback from two key government agencies (i.e., CBO and Foster's Centers for Medicare and Medicaid Services), CLASS supporters introduced a new argument. Garner began referring to a focus group study of more than 20,000 "students" and "young people around the country" that had generated surprising findings which suggested that many of the assumptions underlying the actuarial assessments of CLASS by Foster and the CBO were dead wrong.[32] At an October 2009 Kaiser Family Foundation forum on CLASS, Garner described the first key question put to the students and their response:

Number one, do you honestly think anything—do you have a sense that this is something that's important to you? And what the students reported, which I've often said was a little bit of a surprise to me, and I have seven kids, was yes, they had much more of an appreciation that they may not be who they are 24 hours from now. They have seen lots of kids with car accidents, boogie board accidents; they reported that they had more friends that had Special Ed in school. They were much more exposed to that.[33]

Additionally, Garner announced, this focus group study found that young people were eager to invest in a program like CLASS. "They said yes," Garner reported. The study also found that the students had thought through what type of benefit would be most appropriate. "[T]hey said we need a cash benefit. That way it works for me if I have an accident in a ski resort up in Colorado. And it also works for my family because what they reported when they went home was . . . a lot of conversation about what are we going to do about Grandma. So it was almost as if generationally those conversations began to line up."[34]

At the same event, Larry Minnix, the chief executive officer of LeadingAge, touted the focus group data, too. "We got a problem that 70-percent of the people face and nobody wants to talk about." Nobody, that is, except young people. Minnix continued: "What we found in our focus groups and other things is that younger people, especially, are ready to talk about this and willing to pay because they've seen these issues in their own family."[35]

These remarkable findings flew in the face of conventional wisdom about long-term care—and, for that matter, about what young people are aware of, care about, and want to buy. Yet if the findings were obtained in a methodologically defensible manner and if they were accurately reported by Garner and Minnix, they would suggest that CLASS had a real chance of success. If there was, in fact, a groundswell of young, healthy students clamoring for the opportunity to purchase long-term care insurance, CLASS would have a much higher take-up rate than the number-crunchers at CBO were assuming. As Garner said: "They are the healthy risk pool. They are the individuals who will contribute to a pool for those who need it."[36] Indeed, if the focus group findings reflected reality, it would mean that the actuarial assessments from Foster and the CBO were underestimating CLASS' initial and future enrollment and were therefore inaccurately concluding that the program faced serious fiscal problems. While this study was never released publicly[37] and was not addressed in any of the actuarial assessments, it did play a key role in the public explanation of how and why CLASS came about, and it provided something to point to in the face of an increasing number of skeptical questions about whether enough healthy people would enroll to make the program viable.

On July 22, following the release of a new post-markup version of CLASS, the American Academy of Actuaries released its own report to HELP. The organization praised the committee for adding the Gregg amendment, to what otherwise was an "unsustainable" program. However, the group cautioned that the requirement for seventy-five years of solvency "may not be possible to achieve," and that, without further modifications, CLASS would be insolvent beginning in its eleventh year. Even with modifications, adverse selection could still undermine its viability. However, under an "optimistic" scenario with minimal adverse selection, a $160 average premium might sustain a $75 daily benefit for qualified beneficiaries.[38]

Finally, in November, the CBO responded to a HELP Committee request to score the revised version of CLASS that made it through the markup process. The key figure in the report—$72 billion in savings for the 2010–2019 scoring window—was even better than the CBO's estimate for the earlier version of CLASS. Yet, once again, the report also made clear—at least to anyone wishing to read beyond the $72 billion figure— that the program's budgetary implications after the ten-year window were subject to "considerable uncertainty." The CBO estimated the second decade would also be in the black, but by a much smaller amount. Starting in the third decade, however, CLASS would add to budget deficits "by amounts on the order of tens of billions of dollars for each 10-year period." Even with the seventy-five-year solvency provision, "the CLASS program would inevitably add to future deficits." The report also estimated that the average monthly premium would need to be $123.[39]

In sum, by the fall of 2009, five actuarial assessments were in the mix and had offered somewhat divergent conclusions on CLASS. Richard Foster, from the Centers for Medicare and Medicaid Services in the Department of Health and Human Services, held that CLASS was fundamentally flawed. The HELP Committee had countered with studies by AARP and the Moran Company that ostensibly offered more positive assessments. But Foster pointed out critical differences between CLASS and the types of programs examined in those reports, concluding that they were worthless for assessing the non-mandatory CLASS Act. Finally, the CBO and the American Academy of Actuaries had weighed in, offering, at best, mixed assessments. These reports did, however, suggest that there were potentially viable paths forward involving higher premiums and lower benefits. Yet, the premium levels they identified as necessary for a sustainable program—$123 and $160, respectively—were multiple times larger than the $30 and $65 premiums touted earlier by CLASS advocates.[40] Moreover, they were approaching the premium levels available through private long-term care insurance providers that were widely seen as too expensive—a problem that CLASS was supposedly going to address.

Taken as a whole, the various and varying projections for CLASS point to a fundamental difficulty in the attempts to assess how the program would work. The research base on which these projections were made paled in comparison to what was available for other aspects of health reform. For example, economists like Jonathan Gruber had developed relatively sophisticated and reliable models for health insurance coverage. That kind of research base simply did not exist for CLASS. As a result, neither the program's advocates nor its critics could say with any real confidence how many people would participate in CLASS, what risk profile those individuals would have (i.e., how likely they would be to draw benefits), or what the average premium would need to be. Of course, the CBO and other agencies tasked with making projections are required to come up with precise numbers. Yet lurking behind the apparent precision of premium figures forecast down to the dollar was a considerable amount of educated guessing.

Nonetheless, this largely behind-the-scenes actuarial debate raised profound doubts about CLASS' viability. Even the AARP report trumpeted by CLASS supporters highlighted potentially fatal flaws. And the other study promoted by CLASS activists (i.e., Moran) was based on an inapplicable individual mandate. Retrospectively chronicling this state of affairs two years later, a report issued by a congressional Republican working group alleged that HELP Committee Democrats and administration officials at the Department of Health and Human Services "ignored warnings" and "effectively silenced" Foster.[41] Yet the reports from the CBO and the American Academy of Actuaries—in addition to the focus group study touted by Garner and other CLASS supporters—offered a strained justification for pushing forward. While far from ringing endorsements, CLASS supporters could point to the fact that neither the CBO nor the American Academy of Actuaries explicitly rejected the program outright. Of course, the CBO is not in the business of approving or rejecting programs. Nonetheless, in those generally pessimistic but qualified assessments, there was a rationale for clinging to hope, at least for those desperate to find one. With so many studies and reports—all of which were steeped in tedious and technical details—the water had been muddied. Through a combination of strategy and luck, CLASS supporters could point to those assessments that suggested possible paths forward—however illusory—while ignoring the more obvious take-away conclusion from the multiple reports: CLASS was an unsound policy that had no hope of working in the way its supporters had been claiming, if at all.

CLASS on Capitol Hill, Part 2

A Bipartisan Backlash and the Missing "Fixes"

As summer turned to fall in 2009, CLASS was alive but still very much in limbo. Despite having a foothold in the House bill and having survived the HELP Committee markup, the program faced several procedural hurdles as well as growing resistance in both chambers of Congress.

Perhaps most troubling was a new concession that further undermined the solvency of an already actuarially dubious program. Given the early decision to create a voluntary rather than a mandatory program, the CLASS advocates had then attempted the next best thing for boosting enrollment: an opt-out requirement. That is, rather than relying on people to become aware of CLASS and decide to enroll, early versions of CLASS held that all eligible individuals would be automatically enrolled unless they declined coverage. The opt-out provision carried the political benefit of avoiding a mandate while nudging into the program those individuals inclined to follow the path of least resistance.[1] Like a 401(k) plan, momentum would have been on the side of enrollment and the burden would have been on those seeking to avoid participation. Such a provision would have probably still left CLASS far short of solvency, though it undoubtedly would have boosted participation.

The opt-out provision was eliminated in the fall of 2009 when Senator Herb Kohl (D-WI), purportedly under pressure from private long-term care insurance providers, insisted on an opt-in model. He argued that with an opt-out provision, people would not be aware that they were enrolled. Fearing all could be lost if they refused to accede to the influential Democrat's demand, CLASS supporters capitulated even though they realized the significance of the concession. As one CLASS insider recounted, "we knew right then we'd be in trouble."[2] Indeed, the alteration further weakened a program that, lacking a mandate, was already in serious trouble. Yet no one hesitated to move forward under the opt-in model. From the long-view perspective of CLASS' designers, creating a workable program was not the top objective. Just getting something passed was the key. If that critical goal was accomplished, the program could always be fixed later.

This even weaker version of CLASS now had to survive the procedure of merging the divergent Senate bills reported out of the Finance and HELP committees into a single piece of legislation, a process that would be led by Majority Leader Harry Reid. Then, if CLASS was still standing, it would have to make it through a floor debate and a vote before the full Senate. Each of these steps carried the very real possibility that CLASS could be removed from the health reform package. If it survived, the final step for both CLASS and the Affordable Care Act would be a conference committee in which the versions of health reform passed in the House and the Senate were combined into a single bill prior to a final vote in each chamber. If CLASS managed to advance to the conference committee, it would be all but certain to make it into the final bill sent to the president, although the program could be altered significantly at that last stage.

While the central features of health reform, namely, health insurance coverage, cost containment, and quality of care, continued to command the spotlight, CLASS was garnering more attention. By this point, the cat was out of the bag: Everyone who had given the program any serious thought recognized that, as written, it contained grave actuarial problems that jeopardized its viability.

DISMISSING CLASS: "A PONZI SCHEME OF
THE FIRST ORDER"

As the process of merging the two Senate bills got underway, a new problem for CLASS surfaced: Democrats started attacking the program. This
new split within the party mirrored the divide between the budget-hawk
Democrats serving on Senator Max Baucus' Finance Committee and their
more progressive counterparts on HELP, who were closely linked to the
advocacy groups. On October 23, seven Democratic Senators—Evan Bayh
(IN), Kent Conrad (ND), Mary Landrieu (LA), Joe Lieberman (I-D, CT),
Blanche Lincoln (AR), Ben Nelson (NE), and Mark Warner (VA)—aggres-
sively challenged CLASS in a letter to Reid, urging the Majority Leader to
leave it out of the merged bill. The seven Democratic senators made two
allegations. The first was the familiar charge that CLASS was fundamentally flawed. "While the goals of the CLASS Act are laudable," the group
wrote, "the effect of including this legislation in the merged Senate bill
would not be fiscally responsible. . . . We have grave concerns that the real
effect of [CLASS] would be to create a new federal entitlement program
with large, long-term spending increases that far exceed revenues." The
letter noted that the appearance of savings was deceptive and entirely due
to the five-year pre-benefit period.[3]

The second allegation made by the anti-CLASS Democrats was that the
program's supporters were trying to spend the same pot of money twice.
On the one hand, CLASS supporters were pushing back against the argument that their program was fiscally irresponsible and unviable by saying
that the savings built up during the five-year vesting period would help
pay for CLASS benefits in the years to follow. Yet they were also claiming that CLASS brought huge savings to the larger health reform package,
with the clear implication being that those savings would pay for other
aspects of health reform.[4] The program's supporters, in other words, were
trying to have it both ways. As Senator Nelson pointedly asked a few days
after signing the letter, "How can the money be used to offset the cost of
the legislation and also be set aside to pay benefits? That doesn't make any
sense."[5]

Several days later, Senator Conrad ratcheted up the rhetoric on the double counting allegation. He publicly denounced CLASS as "a Ponzi scheme of the first order, the kind of thing that Bernie Madoff would have been proud of."[6]

Other critics took the double counting allegation a step further by charging that CLASS was a hastily crafted plan inserted into the Affordable Care Act with the explicit goal of distorting the true cost of health reform. "Embedded in the health-care plan," wrote *Fortune* editor Shawn Tully, "is a truly gravity-defying new device: a costly entitlement program portrayed as a way to save money. . . . While no one doubts [CLASS'] humane intentions, its ardent champions have another motive as well." Tully argued that the tens of billions of dollars in Congressional Budget Office (CBO)-projected savings over the first ten years of CLASS not only masked "the disaster lurking just beyond that horizon" for the program itself, but also was a shrewd and cynical ploy to obscure the full cost of Obamacare. In accounting for a major chunk of the Affordable Care Act's alleged savings, CLASS "look[ed] like a gift" to backers of health reform, most of whom were unfamiliar with the program and had zero interest in it beyond its usefulness in making good on their promise that the overhaul of American health care wouldn't cost anything.[7] Likewise, Senator Olympia Snowe (R-ME) charged that "[t]he whole thing was a fiscal masquerade. It was obvious."[8]

Demonstrating savings was indeed absolutely essential for health reform's political viability because the White House and congressional Democrats had made a very public and firm commitment to deficit neutrality. The financial savings that would accompany health reform was a major talking point for its supporters. Not only would health reform improve American medicine, its enthusiasts argued, it would also be a money saver. A typical formulation in December 2009 found President Obama calling health reform "the largest deficit reduction plan in over a decade. . . . And in terms of deficits—because we keep on hearing these ads about how this is going to add to the deficit—the CBO has said that this is a deficit reduction, not a deficit increase. So all the scare tactics out there, all the ads that are out there are simply inaccurate." He further explained: "Now, I just want to repeat this because there's so much misinformation about the cost issue here. You talk to every health care economist out there and they will tell you that ... whatever ideas exist in terms of bending the cost curve and starting to reduce costs for families, businesses, and government, those elements are in the bill." It's unclear how much the president knew about the details of the bill's money-saving "elements" when he uttered these words. But what is quite clear is that CLASS' $72 billion in CBO-certified savings accounted for more than half of the total savings credited to the Affordable Care Act. In other words, CLASS was far and away the most important of what President Obama referred to as "ideas" for "bending the cost curve and starting to reduce costs."[9]

The backlash within the Democratic Party continued in a House caucus meeting when Representative Earl Pomeroy (D-ND) echoed the allegation that CLASS was cobbled together at the last minute simply to make health reform look more economically responsible. He acknowledged that something had to be done about long-term care, but "not some provision cooked up by advocacy groups at the last hour."[10]

This final charge, of course, was largely false. CLASS was anything but a sloppy plan thrown together at the eleventh hour. On the contrary, it had been carefully designed over the course of years and long predated the Obama health reform push.

Yet the program's new critics were by no means entirely off base. Even on its own terms, the CBO-projected savings in CLASS were being double counted, as the letter penned by the Democratic senators pointed out. And while CLASS was certainly not new on the scene, it had been designed with the CBO scoring in mind and with the knowledge that latching onto and appearing to provide money for something like the very health reform legislation then under consideration might well be its only chance of getting to the president's desk.

THE EMERGENCE OF THE "FIXES"

Acknowledging that there was a widening revolt against CLASS and that it did in fact have serious actuarial problems, the lead advocates worked with the HELP committee, officials at the Department of Health and Human Services, the White House, and the Office of Management and Budget to devise a list of potential "fixes." These changes were geared toward limiting eligibility for individuals likely to draw benefits, decreasing benefit commitments, and closing loopholes that allowed for gaming the system. The work requirement, for instance, would have been toughened. As originally put forward, any "working" individual would be eligible for CLASS, and "working" had been defined as earning a minimum of $1,120 annually in three of the previous five years. Under the proposed fixes, individuals would need to make $12,000 in five consecutive years. Likewise, benefits would have been significantly curtailed. Proposed fixes included annual premium increases, slashing the daily benefit after five years or limiting coverage entirely to just a few years, prohibiting those with preexisting conditions that required long-term care from receiving benefits for fifteen years, and starting the daily benefit at $5 or $10 a day for, say, twenty years before it was bumped up to the previously established lower-tier level of $50 a day. And finally, if all else failed, a "failsafe" fix would have granted the Secretary of Health and Human Services the unilateral power to make whatever changes were necessary to ensure that CLASS remained solvent for seventy-five years. Table 6.1 lists the proposed fixes.[11]

While such measures would have certainly helped plug the actuarial holes in the program and given it a much better chance of functioning, they signaled a major retreat on policy grounds. If the fixes were adopted, the resulting program would be vastly different from the one its advocates and supporters had been championing for years. The fixes would have effectively made CLASS subject to the same kind of underwriting that is standard practice in the private insurance market, whereby enrollment qualification and premium levels are based on an assessment of each individual's probability of drawing benefits; those with a high likelihood of becoming benefit eligible pay higher (often much higher) premiums or are denied the opportunity to enroll. This situation is exactly what CLASS—with its lack of underwriting and low premiums—had sought to counter. The fixes would have meant completely shutting out many individuals with disabilities and, for those still allowed to participate,

Table 6.1 PROPOSED FIXES FOR CLASS TO MITIGATE ADVERSE SELECTION, LOWER PREMIUMS, AND INCREASE MARKETABILITY

1. Require employers to inform their employees about CLASS
2. Give the Secretary more flexibility and discretion in determining ADL standards, identifying fraud and abuse, changing premiums, granting exemptions from premium increases, and assessing penalties for missed premium payments
3. Change the work requirement from 3 of 5 years to 5 of 5 years
4. Increase the minimum earnings from $1,120 per year to at least $12,000 per year
5. Allow the Secretary of the Treasury to disclose wage information to the Secretary of Health and Human Services to provide a mechanism for verifying that individuals are working
6. Anti-gaming provisions to eliminate the incentive for individuals to pay premiums for only a short period of time and then rejoin when their health status declines
7. Monthly premium increased annually by a fixed percentage
8. Daily benefit declines by 80 percent after five years
9. Phased enrollment: Initial eligibility restricted to groups with above average health risk profile (e.g., large employers)
10. Enrollees developing ADL limitation resulting from a pre-existing condition would not be eligible for benefits in the first 15 years
11. Daily benefit increases the longer the CLASS policy is held without going into claim
12. Limit the duration of coverage to, for example, 3 years
13. Daily benefit starts low (e.g., $5 or $10) for a fixed time period (e.g., 20 years) before increasing to $50 daily
14. Pre-paid benefit plan
15. Provide authority to conduct an annual study to determine the risk profile of the enrolled population so that the Secretary has more information to consider when setting premium and benefit levels

Table 6.1 CONTINUED

16. "Failsafe: In the [ACA version of CLASS], the Secretary can alter the
    premiums in response to threats to financial stability of the CLASS program.
    However, it is possible the authority in the bill to modify premiums will not be
    sufficient to ensure the program is sustainable. The failsafe provision gives the
    Secretary authority to alter earnings and vesting provisions of the CLASS Act
    to further decrease adverse selection and maintain long-run stability."

ADL stands for "activities of daily living".

SOURCES: U.S. Department of Health and Human Services, "CLASS: Suggested
Technical Corrections," 2010, http://www.thune.senate.gov/public/_files/ClassAct/
ExhibitQ.pdf; U.S. Department of Health and Human Services, "A Report on the
Actuarial, Marketing, and Legal Analyses of the CLASS Program," 2011, http://aspe.
hhs.gov/daltcp/reports/2011/class/index.shtml.

drastically limiting benefit payouts, particularly for individuals who otherwise would have been cashing benefit checks for decades.

Nonetheless, it was increasingly clear to some of the leading CLASS
supporters that their program had come to a fork in the road: These fixes
that substantially watered down the program had to be accepted, or there
would be no program at all. But many of the advocates and groups—
particularly those outside the inner circle—were not so malleable, and
the fixes threatened to unglue the coalition of interest groups, particularly
those representing the disabled community. The drastic alteration that the
fixes represented was summed up by one advocate who, when presented
with a draft of the changes, exclaimed: "You're screwing our people!"[12]

Due to this dissension in the ranks, the fixes were put on ice. "The
[advocacy] groups would have gone crazy" if the fixes had been inserted,
recounted one congressional staffer.[13] Most of the leading figures behind
CLASS who had been part of the Friday Group meetings in Kennedy's
office realized that they would have to make the changes eventually, but
it wasn't worth upsetting the delicate equilibrium of the CLASS coalition
until they had no more room to maneuver.

THE FINAL HURDLES: "THE MONEY SAVED IT, NOT POLICY"

Given the widening split within the Democratic caucus between the budget hawks and the progressives, it was far from certain that CLASS would make it through the merger process and advance to the Senate floor. Yet when Majority Leader Reid unveiled the combined bill on November 19, CLASS had made the cut. The most important factor for its inclusion in the Affordable Care Act was the CBO-reported $72 billion in savings that CLASS brought to the table. According to many individuals interviewed for this project—CLASS supporters and detractors alike—the White House and the Democratic congressional leadership had become increasingly sensitive to cost estimates for health reform, and CLASS' $72 billion in savings represented over half of the Affordable Care Act's CBO-estimated $130 billion in total savings.[14] Consequently, the long-term care program that had been an afterthought for most legislators and the White House during the health reform process had taken on major significance. Regardless of CLASS' long-term economic prognosis, it had become a critical component in making the political argument that health reform would be a money saver.

In the end, then, it came down to the money. As one congressional staffer and strong CLASS supporter put it: "The money saved it, not policy. We needed to pay for the bill. Some were committed to it [on policy grounds], but the money carried the day."[15] To be sure, CLASS maintained a small band of true believers in Congress. But Reid was not among them. His objective was to pass health reform, and CLASS helped by offering savings. Similar sentiments prevailed at the other end of Pennsylvania Avenue. Despite skepticism about CLASS' viability, the White House encouraged its inclusion in the merged bill because of the official savings the program brought to health reform. By this point, of course, everyone knew CLASS' savings were illusory. Yet the CBO projection provided more than enough cover, and Democratic leaders were not going to look their gift horse in the mouth.

Having decided to put CLASS in the combined Senate bill, the merger process afforded a natural opportunity to install some or all of the fixes drawn up by HELP, the Department of Health and Human Services, the White House, and the Office of Management and Budget. Indeed, it was during this merger process that much of the Affordable Care Act's final language and structure were shaped. Yet none of the CLASS fixes were included in Reid's combined bill. Individuals with knowledge of the merger process say that the fixes were left out because of opposition from HELP and the advocacy groups. Those resistant to inserting the fixes correctly recognized that the proposed changes would leave many of "their people" ineligible for CLASS. While some of the advocates reluctantly acknowledged that difficult concessions were going to be necessary at some point, they fought against them and felt no need to compromise until their backs were against the wall. And for those outside of the groups' orbit who were focused on other aspects of the Affordable Care Act, there was certainly no incentive to tinker with CLASS and risk losing its coveted $72 billion in CBO-certified savings. Any necessary changes could wait for the conference committee when health reform was a done deal. So the fixes were once again set aside.

The final hurdle for CLASS came on the Senate floor. For Republicans desperate to kill health reform, CLASS was an easy target that demonstrated the fundamental flaws of Obamacare and called into question the fiscal implications of the entire legislative package. These senators, along with a number of Democrats, hoped to strip the program from the final bill on the Senate floor. On December 4, John Thune (R-SD) offered amendment No. 2901 to do just that. He and Chuck Grassley (R-IA) took the lead in opposing the program during the floor debate. They hammered away at the adverse selection issue and alleged that "[a]dding the ticking time-bomb of yet another unfunded liability to our children and grandchildren through the CLASS Act is irresponsible."[16] They also twice entered into the Congressional Record the October 23 letter penned by the seven dissident Senate Democrats (encouraging Reid to drop CLASS during the merger).[17] Additionally, Thune—stoking the traditional animosity between the aging and disability groups—noted that CLASS' work requirement meant that no current seniors would benefit from the program.[18]

Meanwhile, CLASS supporters accused Republicans of cynically attempting to kill the program as a means to bring down the entire Affordable Care Act. That motivation, they argued, was the only plausible explanation for their boorish behavior, because any lingering concerns over the program's financing had been cleared up thanks to the helpful suggestion from Senator Gregg during the HELP markup. Senator Dodd, for instance, said: "Many of our colleagues have come to the floor in the last few days to claim the CLASS Act will be a long-term drain on the budget. It is not true. Thanks to ... Senator Gregg, the CLASS Act will be required by law to be solvent for 75 years. This was not in our original proposal. It was added in the HELP Committee markup by Senator Gregg, and I thank him for it."[19] Paul Kirk (D-MA) also graciously acknowledged Gregg's contribution: "Let's give proper credit where it is due. With the help of the Republicans on the committee, especially Senator Gregg of New Hampshire, additional safeguards were included to ensure that the act will stand on strong financial footing for years to come.... We credit Senator Gregg for that constructive contribution."[20] Similarly, Senator Harkin (D-IA) expressed gratitude to Gregg for his work in helping to grant Ted Kennedy's dying wish:

> Senator Kennedy worked on this for years. The couple times I talked to him this summer and this spring, this is what he wanted to talk to me about: making sure we included this in the bill. This was his cause.... I ask my friends on the other side of the aisle, why are you against a voluntary program that will enable people to have ... peace of mind? Well, I have heard it said: "Well, maybe the taxpayers will have to pay for this and everything." I will tell you this: In the committee, Senator Gregg—Senator Gregg from New Hampshire, Republican Senator Gregg, my good friend—offered an amendment to make sure the [premium] contributions were the only things that would sustain this program, that it would not become an entitlement.[21]

Shortly thereafter, and not unexpectedly, Harkin's "good friend" joined all the other Republicans in voting for Thune's amendment to eliminate CLASS.

It was less clear how the votes would come down on the Democratic side of the aisle. The seven letter writers were clear ayes, and an unknown number of other caucus members were expected to join them in voting to strip CLASS from the bill. As was the case throughout the lawmaking process, there was "a high degree of uncertainty" about how the votes would fall concerning CLASS.[22] In the end, five additional Democrats—Baucus, Thomas Carper (DE), Claire McCaskill (MO), Mark Udall (CO), and Jim Webb (VA)—joined those who signed the letter to Reid. Thune's amendment to kill CLASS had thus won a 51-47 majority. But because the Senate's unanimous consent agreement for the Affordable Care Act required that amendments garner 60 votes to pass, it was defeated.[23]

CLASS' place in the Senate legislation was now assured.

In staving off the Thune amendment on the Senate floor, CLASS had survived what was perhaps its stiffest challenge. The program's supporters had "been sweating that one" but could now be reasonably confident that CLASS would become a reality, albeit in heavily modified form once the fixes were added in the looming conference committee.[24] But with the Obama administration and top congressional Democrats eager to retain CLASS' CBO-certified $72 billion in savings, the program was a lock to remain in the final package. CLASS had beat long odds to succeed where past proposals had failed. Its champions could rest assured that it would be in the health reform package headed to the president's desk.

THE GREAT UNRAVELING

With legislation passed in both the House and the Senate, the long-elusive health reform overhaul—onto which CLASS had piggybacked—appeared to be a done deal. Only the formality of a conference committee remained.[25] With the heavy lifting over, it was time for a break. The final vote on the Senate bill—in which every Democrat voted "aye" and every

Republican voted "nay"—occurred on Christmas Eve.[26] Congress then went into recess, and staffers were ordered to take several weeks off for the holidays, a welcome respite for the many who had been working seven days a week for months.

Little did they know, however, that it was too early to celebrate. No one saw it coming, but the unimaginable was about to happen in the late Ted Kennedy's Massachusetts.

A Special Election Surprise

Congress reconvened on January 6, 2010, to begin blending the House and Senate legislation in the conference committee. This final stage of the lawmaking process was critical for CLASS because it was the last chance to insert important changes to fix the damage done by crafting a program to meet the imperatives of the CBO scoring regimen. The fixes were a tough pill to swallow for the lead advocates (and some CLASS supporters still strongly opposed them), but there was no other way to square the circle. It was here in the last step of the lawmaking process that CLASS would be transformed from a blatantly unworkable program (though one perfectly tailored to generate CBO-reported savings) into a functional one (even if it would fall well short of its original promises).

At this point, few were paying much attention to the upcoming special election in Massachusetts to fill Kennedy's Senate seat. The Bay State is perhaps the most Democratic in the country, and it was considered a foregone conclusion that Massachusetts Attorney General Martha Coakley, the party's anointed successor to Kennedy, would handily defeat the Republicans' latest sacrificial lamb, state legislator Scott Brown.[27] Prior to serving twelve years on Beacon Hill, Brown had gained minor notoriety as a model. His career in glamour was launched when he graced the pages of *Cosmopolitan* as a nude centerfold, albeit in a demure pose. He later went on to appear, in clothes, on a Times Square billboard and in a photo shoot with Julianne Phillips, one of the era's iconic models. Brown's background in fashion (a profession underrepresented in the contemporary

Congress), may have made "the Cosmo Boy"—as Studio 54's Steve Rubell called him—even easier to dismiss than a standard issue Massachusetts Republican.[28]

While it was a foregone conclusion that Coakley would cruise to victory, that outcome was of the utmost importance in Washington because of the razor-thin partisan breakdown in the Senate that was—with zero margin for error—allowing Democrats to move their agenda without any Republican support. The Democrats held a 60-40 majority in the upper chamber, including the seat held by Kennedy's temporary replacement. With that margin, Majority Leader Reid had just enough votes to block GOP filibusters so long as his caucus was unanimous, as it had been in the Affordable Care Act's Christmas Eve vote and as it would need to be in a final roll call following the conference committee. This meant that even though maintaining Democratic control of Kennedy's seat was all but guaranteed, it was also considered absolutely essential for the health reform process.

For weeks, Coakley's campaign had been perceived as coasting. She gained the Democratic nomination in early December, and then seemed to assume that her ticket to Washington had been punched. Typically, that would be an entirely reasonable assumption in Massachusetts. But this election was unique in more than just its unusual January timing. For starters, Coakley had drawn a more formidable Republican challenger than might have been expected. In his time as a state legislator, Brown had developed a reputation as a moderate, or even liberal, Republican, thereby making him more ideologically palpable to Bay Staters than a typical GOP nominee. And during the short special election campaign, he drove his own pickup from rally to rally to save money, an approach that came to symbolize his everyman credentials and contrasted sharply with perceptions that Coakley was a "limousine liberal" who was too busy measuring the drapes for her new office in Washington to spend time meeting voters on the campaign trail. But perhaps more important than personalities and campaign strategy and tactics, the election was nationalized in that it was held with the health reform process as a backdrop. Brown made the issue the centerpiece of his campaign and promised to be the critical

"41st senator" who would vote to uphold a Republican filibuster of the Affordable Care Act. By early January, polling indicated that Brown had eliminated Coakley's 30-point lead and that the race was a dead heat.[29]

Despite these warning signs, it was only several days prior to the election that the campaign gained significant national attention. At the eleventh hour, with panic setting in at Coakley headquarters, the party called in its A-list stars—including President Obama and former president Bill Clinton—to hit the stump with the fledgling candidate in a last ditch effort to salvage the vital seat. It may have already been too late. By the time Obama and Clinton arrived, Brown was leading in the polls.[30] But if there was any hope of a last second Coakley revival, it was likely squelched four days prior to the election when she committed what amounts to an unforgivable sin in New England. During a radio interview, Coakley scandalously dismissed Brown-supporter Curt Schilling—the Boston Red Sox hero of 2004 "bloody sock" lore—as just "another Yankee fan."[31] In baseball-crazy Massachusetts it was tantamount to mistaking Paul Revere for a Red Coat. The disastrous episode epitomized a hapless campaign.

A few days later, Brown shocked the American political establishment to claim the remainder of Kennedy's term. His victory's connection to the ongoing health reform effort in Washington was impossible to ignore. The *Washington Post* was among many major media outlets pointing directly to health reform as the campaign's definitive issue: "Brown, a little-known Massachusetts state senator 10 days ago, won the special election by running directly against the health-care legislation that Kennedy trumpeted before his August death and that Obama considers his most important legislative priority."[32] *CBS News* was more blunt: "Republican Scott Brown's victory in the Massachusetts Senate special election is a repudiation of President Obama's health care reform package."[33] And it was not simply a symbolic repudiation. The Democrats' loss of their filibuster-proof Senate majority was widely seen as a potential death knell for health reform.[34]

Democrats faced a new reality: their filibuster-proof majority in the U.S. Senate—on which health reform had been predicated—was gone. Even though both the House and the Senate had already voted on and passed comprehensive health reform, final votes were still necessary before the president could sign a bill into law. And now, deprived of their supermajority, Democrats could no longer stave off Republican efforts to hold up the legislation with a Senator Brown–supported filibuster. For many, these facts rendered the 2009–2010 health reform process dead. Yet top congressional Democrats had devised a backup plan. This lifeline for health reform, however, would bring an unanticipated consequence that would, once again, place CLASS in jeopardy.

Reconciliation, the "Byrd Bath," and the Senate Parliamentarian

With the normal conference committee route now unexpectedly blocked, congressional Democrats unveiled their backup plan for health reform. They would use reconciliation, the optional process established by the 1974 Congressional Budget Act, the law designed to impose fiscal restraint and to combat out of control spending. As detailed in chapter 2, reconciliation was originally devised as a way to reduce deficits or increase surpluses by fast-tracking budget legislation by preventing amendments, limiting floor debate, and prohibiting filibusters. For Democrats, utilizing the budget reconciliation process was attractive because it offered a way around the Republican filibuster and thereby permitted legislation to pass through the Senate with a simple majority rather than the normal 60 vote supermajority necessary to stave off filibusters. In the case of health reform, a two-step process would be required. First, the House would pass an identical version of the health reform bill the Senate approved on Christmas Eve. Second, both chambers would pass a separate piece of legislation—known as the "sidecar"—containing all of the changes to the Senate bill that would have been inserted during the conference committee. In the Senate, the rules governing reconciliation would be used to pass the sidecar, depriving the newly bolstered Republican caucus from filibustering. Included in the sidecar package were the fixes for CLASS.

The reconciliation plan allowed Democrats to pass health reform. As such, predictions that Brown's victory would be health reform's kiss of

death proved erroneous. But in forcing the Democrats to use the reconciliation process and the rules governing it, the Massachusetts special election did end up carrying dire consequences for CLASS.

That was because using reconciliation meant abiding by the Byrd Rule.
As explained in chapter 2, the Byrd Rule stipulates that only those proposals with a significant budgetary impact during the scoring window can be
passed via reconciliation. Inevitably, disputes arise about whether something affects the budget sufficiently to be in compliance with this rule.
During the 2009–2010 health reform process, a man named Alan Frumin
had the final say on what was and was not suitable under the terms of
the Byrd Rule. Frumin was the Senate parliamentarian, an obscure and
unelected official that few people beyond Capitol Hill are aware of. The
Office of the Parliamentarian is staffed with experts on the Senate's intri-
cate rules, precedents, and procedures and steeped in the chamber's institutional history, norms, and culture. One does not become the Senate
parliamentarian without having first "apprenticed" in the office for a long
time, usually decades. Parliamentarians are strictly nonpartisan (though
they are appointed and can be fired by the majority leader). They are also
accustomed to working in anonymity. But with the already intense health
reform process entering an unanticipated final phase, the parliamentarian was thrust into the spotlight and received a highly unusual degree of
media attention and public scrutiny.

With health reform now utilizing the reconciliation process, it fell to
Frumin to rule on a myriad of Republican challenges to provisions that
they alleged ran afoul of the Byrd Rule.[35] This process, known as a "Byrd
bath scrubbing," takes place in private before any legislation is brought to
the Senate floor; provisions the parliamentarian deems as failing to meet
the rule's threshold are removed and referred to as "Byrd droppings." As
Senator Gregg said at the time: "He's basically the defense, the prosecu-
tion, the judge, the jury and the hangman in this scenario. It all comes
down to him."[36]

According to individuals involved in the process, following the collapse
of the conference committee, the original set of fixes for CLASS was altered.
At this point, the supporters of CLASS—including some of the executive

branch officials who had helped draft the fixes—were in the awkward position of trying to achieve two different and contradictory goals. First, they had to alter the program enough to make it viable over seventy-five years (in accordance with Senator Gregg's amendment inserted during the HELP Committee markup). Second, they were simultaneously trying to preserve CLASS' CBO-reported savings over the first ten years that were credited to the Affordable Care Act. CLASS supporters concluded that adding the full set of fixes would have meant cutting the CBO-projected savings in half. That is, inserting the fixes that would give the maligned program a chance of succeeding upon implementation would have come at the partial expense of the White House's coveted savings.

At this moment of reckoning, the money won out again. To preserve the savings that had made CLASS attractive to Democratic leaders in the first place, the final set of fixes prepared for the sidecar and presented to the parliamentarian was trimmed down and became more modest in scope than the original set of fixes. Those involved with CLASS were optimistic that they could have their cake and eat it too by inserting just enough changes to both pass muster with the Gregg Amendment's seventy-five-year solvency requirement and keep the ten-year savings. And with a different individual serving as parliamentarian, maybe they could have, because the issues that crossed Frumin's desk were the tough calls that included a considerable amount of gray area.

In a shocking surprise to those who had been working on CLASS and the fixes, Parliamentarian Frumin ruled that the modest set of fixes failed to satisfy the Byrd Rule. That is to say, the savings had been preserved too much. Because the changes for CLASS that were presented to the parliamentarian were so modest, they were deemed as carrying insufficient budgetary implications to satisfy the Byrd Rule. And that rendered them ineligible for the sidecar legislation. Had the full set of fixes been offered, it would have clearly satisfied the Byrd Rule, but it would have eliminated much of the savings CLASS brought to health reform that Democratic leaders wanted to preserve. As a result of the ruling, none of the CLASS fixes made it into the final version of the law. To be sure, CLASS would still move forward to the president's desk. But it would be the unaltered and terribly flawed version of the program that Obama would sign into law as part of the Affordable Care Act.

CLASS supporters thought the parliamentarian made the wrong decision and that the fixes should have been allowed. However, CLASS backers were not the only ones upset with the parliamentarian. In fact, during the reconciliation process, he received far more scorn from opponents of health reform. Senator Orrin Hatch (R-UT), for instance, expressed doubts before any of the Byrd Rule decrees were even handed down. "I'm sure he's a Democrat," Hatch said derisively of the parliamentarian (who, in fact, is a registered independent). "I think he's an honest man, but we'll see." Another Senate Republican, Jim DeMint (SC), was less coy, saying that the parliamentarian was "clearly biased."[37] Away from the relatively decorous Senate, Frumin required police protection in the face of death threats and having his home targeted by Tea Party picketers.[38]

The rancor over the parliamentarian's rulings and the possibility for varying views on the Byrd Rule highlight an inherently imperfect process in which little is clear cut. Yet there is no evidence that the parliamentarian did anything wrong. On the contrary and in keeping with his general reputation as an obsessively nonpartisan honest broker, he seems to have done his job as well as could be expected. Indeed, to the extent there are rules and processes in a complicated institution like the Senate, someone has to interpret them when disagreements arise. The interpreter could, of course, be an elected official or a partisan appointee, but those alternatives to a nonpartisan expert carry their own objections. In Frumin's no-win and unusually high-profile role as Affordable Care Act referee, he made reasonable and defensible, but inevitably controversial, decisions. Like the advocates who designed CLASS, Parliamentarian Frumin was simply following the rules.

FROM THE POLITICS OF LEGISLATION TO THE POLITICS OF IMPLEMENTATION

The lawmaking process was over for CLASS, and in this final scene, the rules of the policymaking system had created chaos once again. This time, there was no backup plan for CLASS. The fixes to take a blatantly unworkable program and give it a chance for success were prohibited by rules established by earlier rounds of good government reforms. As a result, the horribly flawed version of the CLASS Act was pushed along and became law. For health reform supporters and some CLASS advocates, there were arguably some upsides to this outcome. Most importantly, it left the program's coveted CBO-certified savings in place to be factored into health reform's bottom line and to improve the public image of the new law. For some health reform supporters, that was the only thing that mattered. The failure to insert the fixes also offered some relief to those amongst the advocates who had feared that CLASS would be watered down during the conference committee that never occurred.

Yet this conclusion to the policymaking process left CLASS in a precarious and ultimately untenable position. It would be up to the Department of Health and Human Services to attempt to alter and implement the program. But that was problematic because the version of CLASS that got signed into law contained contradictory mandates. The Department of Health and Human Services was now required by law to do the impossible: implement a self-sustaining, optional program that prohibited underwriting in a marketplace with little consumer demand beyond those individuals likely to quickly become benefit-eligible.

CLASS was designed for the politics of legislation, and it succeeded where previous efforts had failed. Yet the policy problem at its core—which had made it politically viable but also threatened its actual functionality—never got resolved during the lawmaking process. Implementing CLASS now appeared to be even more daunting than passing it.

CLASS IS CANCELLED

Nineteen months after the Affordable Care Act's triumphant White House signing ceremony, CLASS' flaws could no longer be ignored. In October of 2011, Health and Human Services Secretary Kathleen Sebelius announced that the Obama administration had been unable to implement this piece of the president's signature legislative accomplishment and was ending its efforts to do so. She explained that "our department has worked steadily to find a financially sustainable model for CLASS. . . . When it became clear that most basic benefit plans wouldn't work, we looked at other possibilities. . . . [W]e cast as wide a net as possible in searching for a model that could succeed. But . . . we have not identified a way to make CLASS work."[39]

Despite the dejected tone of Secretary Sebelius' announcement, the White House appeared unfazed. An unnamed senior White House official—widely believed to be Deputy Chief of Staff Nancy-Ann DeParle, Obama's point person for passing the Affordable Care Act—told *The National Journal* that CLASS "isn't even a hood ornament. It's like the windshield wiper on the back window of a car—but maybe not even that. The CLASS Act is not central in any way to the health care reform act."[40]

While the loss of CLASS may not have bothered the White House, Sebelius' announcement was a crushing blow for the program's committed supporters. Their sense of loss was only made worse by the White House's unexpectedly callous response. Upon learning of the administration official's "windshield wiper" analogy, Connie Garner, the Kennedy staffer and longtime mastermind behind CLASS, said: "That's tough. It was very important to them when it was being debated. I don't know why it isn't important to them now."[41]

Yet there had to be something familiar in the White House official's dismissive attitude. The flippant comment betrayed the sentiments—with roots stretching back decades—of many of health reform's leading progressive supporters: CLASS was dispensable because it had already served its only real purpose. That purpose did not lie in shoring up America's dysfunctional long-term care system, but in generating the appearance of savings to help "pay" for the Affordable Care Act.

Two Can Play at That Game

While the CLASS saga offers a prime example of how the contemporary policymaking rules incentivize the development of deceptive policy, it is far from an anomaly. The tendency for the reform-based rules to perversely shape policy is now built into the system. And though CLASS and the Affordable Care Act were Democratic proposals, Republicans know how to play the game, too. In fact, two of the chief domestic policy successes from the George W. Bush years bear similar hallmarks.

THE BUSH TAX CUTS

Consider first the 2001 and 2003 Bush tax cuts. The president and supporters of these controversial policies framed their legislation as broad-based measures to help average Americans. At the signing ceremony for the 2001 law, for instance, Bush insisted: "We cut taxes for every income-tax payer. We target nobody in; we target nobody out." To drive the point home, he told the story of the Ramos family:

> Steven is the network administrator for a school district. His wife, Josefina, teaches at a charter school. They have a little girl named Lianna, and they're trying to save for Lianna's college education. High taxes made saving difficult. Last year they paid nearly $8,000 in Federal income taxes. Well, today we're beginning to make life for

the Ramos' a lot easier. Today we start to return some of the Ramos' money and not only their money but the money of everybody who paid taxes in the United States of America.[1]

Critics quickly pointed out that while most taxpayers—including the Ramos family—may have received modest benefits, the rich made out like bandits. According to one estimate, for example, 36 percent of the value of the 2001 tax cut was distributed among the wealthiest 1 percent of Americans. By comparison, about the same percentage of the tax cut was divided among the bottom 80 percent of Americans. Furthermore, opponents argued that this massive giveaway to the rich was astonishingly reckless because it caused great harm to the nation's overall economic health and prevented other priorities from being addressed. For instance, ensuring Social Security's long-term viability would have cost less than half of the expected cost of the tax cuts.[2]

Anticipating such objections, the White House, Republicans in Congress, and conservative intellectuals crafted a public rationale for cutting taxes that was predicated on the existence of large budget surpluses during the Clinton presidency. If the government had collected more money from the taxpayers than it required, the argument went, those excess funds should be returned. As Bush commonly put it, "The surplus is not the government's money, the surplus is the people's money." Sometimes he would elaborate. "You see, the growing surplus exists because taxes are too high and government is charging more than it needs. The people of America have been overcharged and on their behalf, I'm here asking for a refund."[3]

The rules that the Congressional Budget Office (CBO) is forced to comply with helped make the Bush administration's case by inflating the extent of the Treasury's overflowing coffers. The CBO is required by law to operate on the current year assumption, meaning that the agency has to proceed as though previously passed taxing and spending dictates will be followed—even in instances where provisions are routinely changed or have little chance of being honored in the future. For example, the CBO had to take seriously the fantasy that popular tax credits and spending programs that were slated to expire would in fact be terminated, even though they were virtually certain to be extended. These faulty assumptions were calculated into the CBO's baseline, giving the illusion of extra money lying around ready to be refunded to taxpayers. Money from the Medicare trust fund was also included in the reported surplus even though members of Congress from both parties had pledged to leave those funds alone. All told, the effect of following accounting rules that were blatantly disconnected from reality greatly inflated the CBO's projection of the surplus. As political scientists Jacob Hacker and Paul Pierson have demonstrated, these faulty budget estimates from the CBO "were a great help" to "the architects of the tax cut [who] designed the proposal to fully exploit them" and then added in "numerous unrealistic assumptions of their own."[4]

The tax cuts themselves were also designed around CBO scoring rules in a way that misleadingly kept the price tag down. Most notably, sunset provisions stipulated that the tax cuts would abruptly end in 2010—prior to the closing of the ten-year budget window—and revert back to their 2001 levels even though the policy designers had every intention and expectation of making the cuts permanent. This design feature meant that cost estimates for the 2001 cuts generated by the CBO and others were based upon a scoring window in which tax cuts were in place for several years followed by a period in which the cuts were entirely eliminated. This structure had the effect of producing a far lower cost projection than if the tax cuts were in place for the full budget window. The CBO, dutifully following the required scoring rules, projected the tax cuts would cost $1.35 trillion. Other projections based on the expectation that the tax cuts would, in fact, be extended placed the total cost at $2.3 trillion.[5]

The 2003 package of tax cuts employed the same trick. This new legislation was officially scored as carrying a cost of $350 billion based on a budget window running from 2004 to 2013. But with only one exception, all of these tax cuts contained sunset provisions that would make them expire somewhere between the end of 2004 and the end of 2008. Once again, the CBO was required to score the legislation as it was written even though it was widely thought that the sunsets would be pushed back or eliminated entirely. If the official score had reflected this far more reasonable assumption, it could have tripled the price tag to as much $1.06 trillion.[6]

Opponents of the tax cuts thought the sunset provisions were particularly galling because the very lawmakers supporting sunsets had made it clear that they planned to make the tax cuts permanent. For instance, promptly following passage of the 2003 package, Republican House Speaker Dennis Hastert (IL) made no effort to conceal his plan to scrap the sunsets: "The $350 [billion] number takes us through the next two years, basically.... But also it could end up being a trillion-dollar bill, because this stuff is extendable."[7] William Gale of the Brookings Institution and future CBO director Peter Orszag argued that employing sunset provisions in this manner "is a serious problem" because it "pushes the nation farther down an already unsustainable fiscal path." They took special note of the strategy employed by Hastert and other supporters of the cuts: "A particularly cynical tendency among some policymakers over the past few years has been to use sunsets to increase the size of the annual tax cut that fits within the multiyear budget constraint, and then subsequently to argue that the sunset must be removed because it creates uncertainty in the tax code."[8]

A key benefit of including the sunsets, then, was to game the cost projection system to hide the real budgetary implications of the tax cuts and to increase their actual size. Moreover, there was good reason to think that the tax cuts would be extended because a trajectory would have been established that would make it politically difficult to avoid extensions as the sunsets approached. Experts at the Center on Budget Policy Priorities, a liberal think tank, denounced "the apparent compliance" with budget targets as "a fiction" and condemned the law's "unprecedented maneuvers." They argued that "once the reasonable assumption is made that these tax cuts continue beyond the sunset date, their costs are seen to explode." Reliance on various "gimmicks," they argued, enabled designers of the tax cuts "to circumvent much of the fiscal discipline the Congressional budget resolution targets [established in the 1974 Budget Act] are supposed to impose."[9]

Other design features worked with the sunsets to set up a political context favorable to extending the tax cuts. The abnormal use of phase-ins, for instance, made some of the tax cuts take effect slowly, with the bulk of the rebate coming at the end of the scoring window. This policy design at once reduced the total cost of the tax cuts, while also gradually raising expectations among Americans that they would be paying increasingly lower taxes.[10]

Time proved the critics right when it came to extending the tax cuts. Most of the Bush tax cuts were made permanent in 2012.

Ultimately, the CLASS program and the Bush tax cuts featured different players and took place in different policy arenas, but the symmetries are striking. In a blistering, multifaceted assault on the Bush tax cuts, Hacker and Pierson argue that the legislation only passed because of "the capacity of political elites ... to manipulate the reception of their proposals through ... policy design. Central features of [the legislation] cannot be explained without taking into account how policymakers highlighted some benefits and actions, while obscuring or disguising others." They go on to conclude that "[t]he legislation was loaded with features that make little sense as tax or economic policy, but tremendous sense for the purposes of political manipulation."[11] If the final sentence of their critique was tweaked by swapping the word "health" for "tax," one could easily imagine it being uttered about CLASS by one of its strident critics.

MEDICARE PART D

Another marquee domestic policy accomplishment from the George W. Bush presidency is also instructive. Prior to Bush's election in 2000, rising drug costs had drawn fresh attention to the prescription drug gap in Medicare coverage. During his first presidential campaign, the Texas governor pledged to propose an addition to Medicare that would provide prescription drug coverage for American seniors. And though his first years in office were consumed by the tax cut debate and the response to the September 11 terror attacks, Bush turned his attention to Medicare expansion in 2003. In his State of the Union Address in January of that year, the president called for a new prescription drug benefit within Medicare and set a price ceiling for this new program at $400 billion over its first ten years.[12] The result was the Medicare Modernization Act of 2003, which created Part D of Medicare to cover prescription drugs for senior citizens. It was the largest expansion in the program's history. The bill had been aggressively championed by the White House and was passed by Republican congressional majorities in the face of broad opposition from Democrats.

The CBO estimated the program's ten-year cost to be $395 billion, leaving it just shy of Bush's ceiling.[13] But that figure did not mean the new program's costs would be proportionately divided over the coming decade. Instead, like CLASS, it represented a heavily back-loaded program. The first two years combined would cost just over $1 billion before jumping to $26 billion for year three and then $39 billion in year four, when the program would be fully implemented. From there, costs would continue to climb dramatically each year until they reached $73 billion in year ten. Beyond the ten-year window, it was expected that annual costs would continue their steep climb and that expenses for the second decade would exceed $1 trillion.[14] In short, the program's design was ideal for generating a politically satisfactory CBO score. And the agency's $395 billion cost estimate was quite advantageous in making the Medicare expansion more politically palpable even if it was profoundly unhelpful in gauging the true cost of the new prescription drug benefit.

The White House and Republican leaders needed all the help they could get. Even with the attractive cost estimate, the bill escaped the GOP-controlled House of Representatives by the slimmest of margins and only after a highly unusual extension of the voting period during which the leadership and Vice President Dick Cheney pressured recalcitrant Republicans to switch their votes. Further evidence of the importance of the CBO's estimate came to light shortly after Bush signed the bill into law when news broke that the administration had suppressed its own in-house cost estimate showing a much higher price tag. The president's Office of Management and Budget had determined, using a different set of assumptions than the CBO, that the bill would cost not $395 billion, but $534 billion.[15] Evidence from emails—later supported by testimony before the House Ways and Means Committee—indicated that a key executive branch official involved in that scoring process had been ordered to with-hold from Congress anything indicating a price tag in excess of Bush's stipulated $400 billion and was warned that "the consequences for insub-ordination are extremely severe."[16] Had the alternative cost projection been known, the bill would never have arrived on the president's desk.

"Good government" reforms undertaken in the 1970s have introduced a new set of biases into the policymaking process. The ramifications of these reforms have been wide ranging. One key outgrowth has been that American governing institutions now operate in a manner that allows—even encourages—the willful manipulation of the CBO's all-important system of cost estimating. In other words, the rules developed to block bad policies have actually created a new set of incentives that can lead directly to the very thing they were designed to prevent. Everybody's doing it.

Conclusion

The mystery at the heart of the CLASS saga isn't why the Obama administration abandoned it. The real puzzle is how—despite its obvious design flaws, despite opposition from many of health reform's most prominent liberal supporters, despite the American political system's steep hurdles for passing anything, despite how partisan politics works, and despite the rules in place to specifically protect against this kind of legislation—CLASS became law in the first place.

More than anything else, CLASS was a product of the institutional rules governing contemporary policymaking. The very reforms designed to make the policymaking process in Congress more economically credible and accountable created an institutional framework that encouraged the development of this defective policy and made it a politically essential add-on to the Affordable Care Act. Understanding how and why CLASS was designed in such a problematic manner, moved through a resistant Congress, and helped ensure passage of the most important social policy legislation in decades provides insight into how the policymaking process actually works, quite apart from standard textbook accounts.

LEARNING FROM FAILURE

Long-term care's policy history contained lessons that were internalized by CLASS' designers. In interviews, advocates who designed CLASS spoke directly and often about these lessons, all of which pointed to a policy area with severe political constraints. An awareness of these constraints gleaned from past failures helps to explain what otherwise appear to be incomprehensible design features. CLASS was not a misguided plan grounded in naiveté, but rather a sophisticated attempt to do something—anything— about a marginalized policy area in crisis. If the program as originally proposed and passed proved to be unworkable, which was certain, its designers anticipated that it could be revised at the last stage of the lawmaking process or through bureaucratic discretion under the safety of formal law.

In this way, the CLASS Act's flawed design is best understood in the context of political learning grounded in long-term care's policy history. CLASS was designed to overcome the political hurdles that had thwarted all previous attempts to create a national long-term care program. In the decades prior to the 2009–2010 health reform process, long-term care proponents had suffered a string of failed attempts to enact a national program. These failures did not alter their ideas about which policy reforms or proposed solutions were preferable; CLASS advocates certainly would have preferred the kind of social insurance programs proposed in previous attempts at reform. Rather, CLASS was informed by political learning grounded in what political scientist Aaron Wildavsky has referred to as a "strategic retreat."[1] In a process of political learning based on earlier failures, the framers of CLASS determined that their dream of a social insurance program would be a political nonstarter. Political viability required a program that was both self-sustaining and optional. While this was an unpleasant realization, those stipulations appeared to be the price for having any chance of achieving a national program. CLASS' key architects were willing to pay that price, and they set out to craft a policy structured around those requirements. If they succeeded in passing it into law, they thought it would provide a critical foothold and set the stage for something bigger and better. Thus, they consciously developed a new framework for a national program that was designed to facilitate political acquiescence at those points where earlier proposals had met terminal resistance.

The CLASS case deviates from standard conceptions of learning through failure. The concept of learning is typically used to emphasize how established policy generates feedback effects that influence future policy decisions. This scholarship includes learning through failure, but generally only in the sense of fully implemented policies that come to be seen as failures. The learning process for CLASS, on the other hand, was grounded in learning tactical lessons based on repeated political failures to enact a long-term care program over the course of several decades. As such, the CLASS case helps to advance our understanding of political learning by demonstrating how failed efforts to enact policy can be just as influential in shaping future policymaking efforts as other forms of political learning.

The process of political learning that informed CLASS' design yielded a remarkable success for the program's supporters: CLASS managed to make it through the lawmaking process and get signed into law. Yet in crafting a politically viable program, the designers of CLASS sacrificed sound policy. To be sure, political viability is important for moving a program from the drawing board and into law. But now, following the CLASS Act's collapse, it is abundantly clear that while addressing political constraints may be necessary, it isn't sufficient.

THE CLASS ACT AS A WINDOW INTO POLICYMAKING IN THE POST-REFORM CONGRESS

The CLASS saga also sheds light on how the contemporary American political system's policymaking process operates in a more general way. The rise and fall of the CLASS Act adds to our understanding of policy failure and illuminates how government really works in practice by showing why unsound policies get developed and how they can become law despite the many safeguards designed to filter out flawed policy proposals. In the case of CLASS, then, some features of the American political system that are designed to prevent flawed policy failed to do so, while others actually incentivized and encouraged the development of the very thing they are supposed to prevent.

The American political system was designed to prevent the enactment of bad policy. As James Madison explained in Federalist No. 51

and Federalist No. 62, the preservation of liberty was a central task in designing the Constitution and the "provision for [its] defense must in this, as in all other cases, be made commensurate to the danger of attack." Clearly Madison and his fellow constitutional framers perceived considerable danger because the political system they put into place contained an elaborate set of "auxiliary precautions" and "impediments . . . against improper acts of legislation" and "schemes of usurpation."[2] Over time, even more veto points have been incorporated into the political system, particularly in Congress.[3]

It is well worth considering the numerous points at which CLASS could have and, by the design of the American political system, should have been stopped. One of these is the Madisonian conception of pluralism in which interests counter interests. Many interests held a stake in the 2009–2010 health reform process, the vast majority of which were resistant to the inclusion of any long-term care program. Many viewed long-term care as a liability that could drag down and jeopardize the entire health reform process, as some allege happened during the Clinton reform effort in the 1990s. Others were resistant to the CLASS Act on its own terms. And while the program's supporters in Congress were unusually influential and serendipitously occupied key committee posts, they were few in number. Yet, somehow, the other interests failed to marginalize CLASS and instead allowed two natural antagonists—the disability and aging lobbies—to work together to move the program into the Affordable Care Act.

Congressional safeguards seemingly should have stopped CLASS, too. The textbook explanation of how a bill becomes a law posits that an early step in the process includes passage by the relevant committee in each chamber. One of the advantages of the committee system is that it divides tasks among legislators according to expertise. As a result, before a bill gets considered by the full House or Senate, it has to pass muster with those lawmakers who know the most about that type of legislation. Normally a program like CLASS would have to go through the Senate Finance Committee and the House Ways and Means Committee. These two "money committees" are charged with keeping the nation's fiscal house in order, and the members approach programs like CLASS with an eye toward ensuring that the numbers add up. During the 2009–2010 health reform process, members of these committees and their chairmen were known opponents of CLASS. Once again, these institutional norms suggest CLASS should have been stopped in its tracks or forced to endure heavy modifications.

Finally, CLASS might have been expected to collapse in the face of scrutiny from the Congressional Budget Office (CBO). The agency was founded to provide Congress with analysis of proposed programs, and its scoring process is designed to offer accurate assessments of the fiscal implications of pending legislation and to alert Congress to potential problems. Yet CLASS not only survived but thrived after the CBO released reports saying it would save tens of billions of dollars.

Pushing against these institutional hurdles were several forces that propelled CLASS into law. First, the program managed to evade the hostile congressional committees it would have typically faced. On the Senate side, the unusual power and influence of Edward Kennedy and his position as chair of the Committee on Health, Education, Labor, and Pensions (HELP) was critical. Without Kennedy's stature and influence, which even loomed over health reform when he was on his deathbed in Massachusetts, it is inconceivable that CLASS would have made it through the legislative process. Among other things, CLASS was allowed to bypass the Finance Committee and proceed exclusively through HELP, a highly unusual evasion of standard committee procedure. On the other side of Capitol Hill, the House Energy and Commerce Committee—home to CLASS sponsor Frank Pallone, Pepper Commission veteran Henry Waxman, and all-around long-term care champion John Dingell—wanted to demonstrate House-side support for the program. But to do so, they had to circumnavigate the hostile Ways and Means Committee, through which any legislation with revenue implications had to pass. Despite the obvious revenue implications CLASS carried, the program's supporters on Energy and Commerce eluded Ways and Means by creating a "shell"—a version of the program that was devoid of financing provisions. In so doing, CLASS' small band of House supporters demonstrated—at least to the casual observer—that the program had support in the lower chamber. In short, the small but well-placed cohort of Senators and Representatives who supported CLASS worked hard to evade the two "money committees" with expertise in and responsibility for overseeing programs like CLASS because those committees were opposed to it. Their success in doing so demonstrates the importance of having experienced and influential legislative champions.

Another help to CLASS' advancement was that the comprehensive health reform backdrop provided something of a smokescreen. The program had failed to find traction in earlier sessions of Congress as a stand-alone measure. But with attention focused on the big ticket issues of health reform, CLASS was allowed to move forward in relative anonymity and without too much attention being focused on the program. The larger process also allowed CLASS to survive its only direct vote in either chamber of Congress despite a majority voting against it. Due to the supermajority threshold in place for adding amendments to the health reform bill on the Senate floor, the 51-47 majority voting in favor of an amendment to remove CLASS was insufficient to do so. Typically, the burden falls on those trying to move legislation forward in the Senate, where supermajorities are usually required. But the only direct vote CLASS encountered was one in which the burden fell on those attempting to halt forward momentum.

Finally, the most important reason CLASS moved forward was because it was designed to conform to the new rules of the policymaking process that were established under the 1974 good government reforms. One outgrowth of these reforms has been to unintentionally institutionalize a system in which policymakers are incentivized to design economically unsound programs.

CLASS was perfectly designed to use the rules of the new policymaking system to its own advantage, particularly those surrounding the all-important CBO scoring process. By creating a program that only collected premiums (i.e., paid out zero benefits) for a full half of the CBO's standard ten-year scoring window, CLASS managed to appear to be a financial windfall. In reality, CLASS' "savings" were illusory. Once CLASS started paying benefits, it was clear that the program, as it was described and as it appeared on paper, would become unsustainable. And while the CBO, among many others, noted this problem, the most important aspect of the agency's reports is the numerical cost projection. CLASS' widely lampooned design flaws, then, were attributable not to naïve idealism, but instead to a carefully crafted legislative strategy.

CLASS' designers attempted to shoot the moon—and they won, at least initially, by getting their program attached to the Affordable Care Act. The triumph of CLASS in not only evading a debilitating CBO score, but actually manipulating the process to give off the appearance of savings, was absolutely central to its inclusion in the Affordable Care Act. More important than demonstrating the appearance of viability for the program itself, the CBO score made CLASS an asset to the larger health reform process because it accounted for more than half of the Affordable Care Act's total savings. This was more than sufficient for the White House and the congressional leadership to insist on keeping it in the bill despite widespread knowledge of CLASS' problems toward the end of the lawmaking process. In the larger context of health reform, the purported CLASS savings were important in making the public case for the Affordable Care Act, and thereby in facilitating passage of what is arguably the most important social policy legislation since Medicare and Medicaid were created.

Yet CLASS' designers' adroit use of the policymaking rules was upended by other rules just as they were attempting to play it straight and correct their flawed policy. Fixes were drafted and ready to be inserted into the final legislation during the conference committee. But after Republican Scott Brown claimed Kennedy's Senate seat in a special election, that plan was no longer viable and Democrats had to turn to the reconciliation process, which is governed by the Byrd Rule. The key player in enforcing the Byrd Rule is the parliamentarian, an unelected and—outside of the Senate—unknown official. In a controversial decree, the parliamentarian ruled that the CLASS fixes failed to satisfy the standards of the reconciliation process. The ruling meant that the effort to fix the damage done by the need to satisfy the imperatives of the CBO scoring process was upended by yet another rule designed to prevent bad policy.

IMPLICATIONS FOR THE POLICYMAKING PROCESS
AND AMERICA'S SOCIAL WELFARE STATE

The CLASS Act's rise and fall carries important lessons about how policy gets made in the contemporary American political system. The first lesson is that the system's numerous safeguards, which were designed to prevent unsound policy, now serve to incentivize and reward its development. This is particularly apparent with regard to the important role played by the CBO. Born of the 1974 Congressional Budget and Impoundment Control Act, the CBO is tasked with offering unbiased assessments of the fiscal implications of pending legislation and to alert Congress to potential problems. The scores produced by the CBO indicating how much a proposed new program will cost or save have become a central feature of the policymaking process. The CBO does remarkable work but is constrained by rules that are now routinely gamed, making a mockery of the cautious, responsible scrutiny that the agency's work is supposed to provide.

Progressive champions of health reform may be inclined to shrug dismissively at any kind of process-based concern associated with passage of the Affordable Care Act or to see it as an entirely acceptable trade-off for achieving a long-sought goal. However, the Bush tax cuts should serve as a cautionary tale and a reminder that a different Congress working with a different president could exploit the same rules for less salutary and noble purposes.

It is also worth bearing in mind that CLASS, the Bush tax cuts, and the Medicare prescription drug law are far from comprehensive in cataloging the opportunities for members of Congress to abuse the CBO scoring process to make legislation look better than it actually is. For instance, an alternative tactic is an "advance appropriation," in which legislators appropriate money but dictate that it cannot actually be dispensed until the next fiscal year. The CBO scores bills based on when money actually leaves the Treasury, not based on when it is appropriated. As a result, legislators can spend money on projects while also claiming to be fiscally responsible based on the CBO's score.

Another heavy-handed method is by "directed scorekeeping," in which Congress can dictate to the CBO how to score a particular bill. Congress can, simply by writing instructions into the legislation, suppress the costs or exaggerate the benefits of a particular bill, and the CBO must comply. Directed scorekeeping can have some benefits in that it allows Congress to direct the CBO to account for certain factors that it otherwise would ignore. But the risk for abuse is strong. Dan Crippen, the CBO director during the Clinton administration, has said that the adjustments mandated by Congress shifted the CBO's projections under him by "$17 billion for the House and $16 billion for the Senate."[4] And while the CBO typically notes the impact of the adjustments in its analysis, its official estimate must reflect the wishes of Congress.

Certain legislative moves could make it harder to manipulate the CBO scoring rules. Senators Russ Feingold (D-WI) and George Voinovich (R-OH) sought to address manipulations of the CBO's ten-year scoring window with the Truth in Budgeting and Social Security Protection Act. They introduced the measure in three consecutive Congresses beginning in 2002, though it never became law. Their proposal called for the CBO to estimate costs over a twenty-year window and determine if expenditures in the second decade will grow by 150 percent or more. If they did exceed that threshold, a supermajority vote would be required before the legislation proceeded.[5] The bill has withered in recent years, but a reform effort along these lines still holds appeal. Another compatible possibility would be to establish restrictions on backloaded spending. Like the Feingold-Voinovich measure, a threshold could be identified at which year-to-year discrepancies were disallowed unless an affirmative supermajority vote overruled the limitation. Directed scorekeeping and advance appropriations could be similarly constrained.

To be sure, these kinds of reforms carry their own limitations. Efforts to prevent gaming the ten-year budget window, for instance, would necessitate an unavoidable degree of arbitrariness about where lines are drawn, and any new threshold could potentially be used to shape policy in the same way current rules have done so. Moreover, cost estimating ten years out is hard enough; extending that window would only make the CBO's job more challenging and render its projections less reliable because the farther one looks into the future, the higher the degree of uncertainty. But despite these difficulties, reforms along these lines would make brazen manipulations of the CBO considerably more difficult and increase transparency in how policies are constructed.

The CLASS case also underscores a broader and troubling feature of the contemporary American welfare state and its relationship to the policymaking process. Having evolved over many decades, the welfare state is now both recklessly lavish and pettily cruel. It overcompensates in some areas and, partially as a result, overlooks issues posing the greatest threats to today's middle class. When it comes to programs initiated decades ago, the welfare state can appear carelessly generous. The richest Americans over the age of sixty-five, for instance, still receive massive government assistance in the form of a public pension and government-subsidized health care even as the programs providing these benefits face long-term fiscal challenges. But when it comes to problems like long-term care that have emerged more recently and pose real burdens—financial and otherwise—the American welfare state can be downright miserly. Ideas seeking to address these newly emergent social challenges are held to a standard that their predecessors never faced and could never have satisfied. Yet efforts to modernize these old programs face impenetrable resistance.

Part of the difficulty in addressing new problems can be traced to the "fiscalization" of policy debates. Following the era of congressional reform, policy debates in the United States have, as political scientist Eric Patashnik has explained, become increasingly fiscalized, meaning that "programs are routinely debated not in terms of their substantive merits but rather of their budgetary impact." This shift has drastically altered the type of policies that can be successful, the strategies used to advocate for them, and the political context in which they are considered. Under this altered legislative environment, as Paul Pierson has noted, "[t]he main road to new policy" now leads through the budget. "Politicians aspiring to produce 'change' must first confront the deficit." [6] In other words, proposals for new programs have enormous hurdles to overcome if they aren't revenue neutral or money savers. Even if there's a legitimate, demonstrated need, money rules the day.

The fiscalization of health policy was on clear display throughout the 2009–2010 health reform process, beginning with the president's commitment to deficit neutrality. But perhaps more than anything else, it was the CLASS Act that highlighted the extent to which the process was fiscalized. In the public debate over CLASS, attention focused almost exclusively on whether it would save or cost money. Virtually no interest was shown in assessing the extent to which CLASS represented a sensible approach to addressing a major problem. Even when the bubble burst and the program's real costs came into focus, attention centered strictly on fixing it, which meant making it deficit neutral. Committing new resources on behalf of a worthwhile program was simply not part of the discussion.

At the same time as policy debates over new programs have become increasingly fiscalized, preexisting programs have become resistant to change even as demographic shifts have suggested that reforms are necessary. In 1940, when Social Security was fully implemented, the life expectancy of people reaching the age of sixty-five (and thus, qualifying for the program's full benefits) was seven years less than it is today. A reform in the early 1980s sought to address this new reality, but only initiated a process to slowly raise the retirement age to sixty-seven over twenty-two years. Even more challenging is the change in the ratio of active workers to retirees receiving a pension. In 1960, there were 5.1 workers per beneficiary, but by 2005 there were only 3.3. By 2060, projections indicate that there will be only two active workers for each beneficiary.[7] Medicare has similar issues. There are obvious solutions to shore up these pillars of the welfare state, including raising the retirement age and progressively indexing benefits to reduce payments and subsidies to the wealthiest seniors. But there is a reason why Social Security is known as the third rail of American politics: even these kinds of modest and sensible proposals face enormous political challenges. By clinging to these programs as they currently exist and resisting any modernizations, the nation's capacity to address new challenges is compromised.

Perhaps foremost among these new challenges facing middle-class America is long-term care. The nation's current approach to addressing it is to leave frail seniors and the severely disabled to fend for themselves. Medicaid does offer a safety net, but eligibility for assistance through the program requires impoverishing oneself. This arrangement hits the various socioeconomic segments of the country differently. Those with ample resources and sufficient wealth to self-fund their care are often shielded. And the transition to Medicaid is less of a jolt to those with few assets at stake to begin with. But for a large majority of Americans, financing long-term care is often economically ruinous. Moreover, the current arrangement works poorly and poses grave problems for state budgets.

In short, the American political system appears unable to address new challenges or reform a long-existing set of privileged programs. Exacerbating this problem are the technocratic abuses of the policymaking system that stunt the nation's ability to adapt to changing circumstances by pushing policymakers to craft policies that purportedly offer all of the gain with none of the pain.

IMPLICATIONS FOR THE FUTURE OF LONG-TERM CARE IN AMERICA

There is a tragic element to the story of the CLASS Act and it is a familiar one to the advocates who have dedicated their lives to the individuals and families struggling with long-term care. It is a story that should also help sharpen our understanding of the challenges inherent in confronting long-term care and draw into focus the range of potential reforms.

Is There Any Way CLASS Could Have Worked?

From beginning to end, something of a disconnect existed between CLASS' supporters and its detractors because, to a degree, the two camps were talking about different things. The critics looked at CLASS as it appeared on paper, as it had been described by its supporters, and as it was analyzed by the CBO and Richard Foster, the Medicare actuary. From this perspective, CLASS was indeed an unworkable program. Notwithstanding any minor critiques of the methodology employed by the CBO and Foster, there was no reasonable hope that the program—as it had been described and as it was written—could function in a sustainable way.[8] Eventually even CLASS' principal advocates tacitly acknowledged as much with the drafting of the fixes.

And yet, to its leading supporters, CLASS was conceptualized—at least toward the end—much more broadly. CLASS never hinged on this or that premium or daily benefit figure. CLASS was better understood as a new idea for approaching long-term care in a more humane and cost efficient manner. As such, CLASS' critics were unreasonably hung up on the program's fine print and too dismissive of the basic concept. Critics failed to recognize CLASS' flexibility; if it didn't work as written, it could simply be adjusted by the Secretary of Health and Human Services. The program's supporters insist that if it had gone through the full legislative process—if the fixes had been included—and if the secretary had been given the power to alter the program on an as-needed basis, then CLASS would have worked.

From this perspective, it is amazing and heartbreaking to realize how close CLASS came to being a reality. While there were many missed opportunities to place the CLASS fixes into the health reform legislation, it is nonetheless true that if Martha Coakley's campaign to retain Kennedy's Senate seat for the Democrats had avoided being the improbable disaster that it was, CLASS would have become law with the benefit of the fixes. It proves the old saying that elections have consequences. CLASS was a casualty of this one.

Even after failing to get the fixes passed as law through reconciliation, many CLASS supporters argued that Secretary Sebelius still had the legal power to administratively alter the program on her own. They maintain it was a political decision to drop CLASS and suggest that the White House buckled amidst the array of other implementation challenges facing the Affordable Care Act, such as the legal battle over the individual mandate for health insurance. Some of the advocates place the blame squarely on

Nancy-Ann DeParle, the White House point person on health reform and the presumed source quoted in the press as disfavorably comparing CLASS' importance to that of a car's hood ornament. Referring to her as "an evil witch," albeit one with "nice shoes," one prominent advocate insisted that "if it hadn't been for Nancy-Ann, it would have worked."[9] That perspective may be excessively influenced by anger and frustration over DeParle's dismissive attitude, because others closer to the implementation process maintain that she was never out to get CLASS, only that she (like her boss) prioritized other things. In any event, there were widely differing opinions within the administration over the extent of Sebelius' authority to administratively alter the program. And the last minute efforts by CLASS supporters to insert the fixes legislatively suggest that they knew that making the changes administratively was dicey.

Taking CLASS supporters on their own terms, two questions emerge that are important to the story of their program and for thinking through its lessons for future reform efforts. First, would CLASS have actually worked if the fixes had made it in? And second, if it would have worked, what would this functional version of CLASS have looked like in practice?

To start with, would CLASS have been viable with the fixes? Maybe. Tellingly, even the program's leading advocates weren't sure. Writing shortly after the Affordable Care Act became law and long before the administration gave any hint of abandoning it, Barbara Manard, a key CLASS advocate, concluded an essay defending the program on a revealing note. "Will CLASS work?" she asked. Her answer: "No one knows. It hasn't been tried before."[10]

A study of CLASS released shortly after it became law highlighted the challenge. Alicia H. Munnell and Josh Hurowitz, two scholars at the Center for Retirement Research at Boston College, concluded that CLASS "faces enormous challenges" and that "without adjustments, adverse selection will create a death spiral of rising premiums and declining participation." The changes they identified were in line with the fixes that failed to get inserted into the legislation. "However," they conclude, "even if all of these suggestions are adopted, premiums may never reach an affordable level for middle-class households."[11]

Undoubtedly, the fixes would have given CLASS a much better chance at viability because they were effectively ways of introducing underwriting. In this way, they would have directly helped to mitigate the program's severe adverse selection problem because those most likely to draw benefits would not have been allowed to enroll in the first place.

Key officials well versed in the economics of health policy implementation at the Department of Health and Human Services were confident that with these kinds of measures, and with sufficient flexibility to adjust the program going forward, CLASS could have operated in a self-sustaining manner. By no means does that suggest that CLASS would have been a wild success, only that it would have met its legal obligation to be self-sufficient over seventy-five years.

Yet the Munnell and Horowitz study drove home one reason for uncertainty about whether there was any way for the fixed version of CLASS to work. Unlike the fairly reliable models for standard health insurance that informed the Affordable Care Act's creation, there was little confidence behind the assumptions that went into the actuarial assessments of CLASS. Neither the program's supporters nor its detractors could confidently predict how many people would enroll, the risk profile of those enrollees, or the average premium necessary to maintain CLASS. Estimates of these absolutely central variables were wide-ranging, and the ramifications of the assumptions made by those examining CLASS greatly influenced overall assessments of the program. For instance, Munnell and Hurowitz began by assuming a generous 6 percent enrollment (as compared to the CBO's estimate of 3.5 percent, Richard Foster's 2 percent, and lead CLASS advocate Connie Garner's 5 percent).[12] Even with that comparatively optimistic assumption, they found that under a most likely, or base case, scenario, CLASS' average monthly premium would be $194, which is slightly higher than those available in the private market. A more optimistic scenario for CLASS yielded a $121 premium. But under an entirely plausible scenario in which enrollees were heavily skewed toward those aged forty and over, a prohibitive average premium of $312 would be necessary.[13]

Assume for the moment, though, that it was possible to make CLASS functional. What would this workable version of the program have looked like? Including the fixes would have severely eroded the original idea behind CLASS. From the beginning, CLASS was touted as a program that would be open to nearly all Americans and that it would offer an affordable alternative to plans available in the dysfunctional private insurance market. In practice, a potentially workable version of CLASS would never have been able to come anywhere close to meeting those benchmarks. Lacking mandatory participation or outside subsidies, many people would have been denied the opportunity to enroll, and the people shut out would have been those most in need. Implementing CLASS with the fixes, then, would have been a profound disappointment for much of the sprawling coalition behind it because doing so would have violated the essence of the program as it was understood by its grassroots supporters.

CLASS' leading advocates claim that even with the fixes, their program would have still held comparative advantages against plans offered by private insurers. For starters, CLASS supporters argued that as a public option, there would be no need to make a profit, and consumers would have more faith that the government would honor its commitment than a private insurance company. Another comparative advantage was that benefits under private plans typically last only several years as compared to CLASS' lifetime coverage. Had the lifetime benefit remained in place after the fixes (which is far from certain), it would have been especially helpful to younger individuals with disabilities. But other design features probably would not have worked to CLASS' advantage. For instance, CLASS would have offered only about half as much money per day in benefits as private plans. Likewise, premium comparisons might have hurt CLASS. As the Munnell and Horowitz analysis laid bare, comparing CLASS' premiums to those on the private market is challenging. However, speaking very roughly, premiums under a heavily modified and potentially workable CLASS program almost certainly would not have been much lower than those available on the private market, and they might have been much higher. A final design difference that would have worked to CLASS' disadvantage in the eyes of comparison shoppers was its five-year vesting period. Taken cumulatively, CLASS had a clear comparative advantage for disabled individuals expecting to live long lives because of the lifetime benefit (again, under the questionable assumption that some version of this provision would have remained in place). But for older individuals, the more modest daily benefit combined with the five-year vesting period probably would have been less attractive than private market offerings.

In sum, it is possible that CLASS could have functioned if the fixes and other adjustments had been made, though we will never know for sure. Yet even if a program operating under the name of CLASS had proven sustainable, it would have been much more modest and served a much more restricted population than the one originally envisioned, described, and introduced as legislation.

The Limited Range of Options

The CLASS experience draws into sharp relief the limited range of options currently available for addressing long-term care. The political context is central to reform, and this realization constituted a great strength of the advocates who designed CLASS. To their frustration, the advocates recognized that they were constrained by a lack of public demand for long-term care reform. In addition to the American public's ignorance and misinformation concerning long-term care, sociologist Sandra Levitsky has argued that ideas for reform also run counter to the powerful and pervasive "ideology of family responsibility." That is, Americans, including caregivers, believe it is the natural duty of family members, rather than the state, to care for their relatives.[14] As a result of these factors, no groundswell of demand for additional government intervention has appeared. And the lack of public demand only reinforces the aversion to any program with mandatory participation or lacking deficit neutrality. Simply put, this was the disadvantageous political reality within which the advocates of CLASS were forced to craft their policy. The lead advocates recognized these constraints and were attempting to make whatever progress was possible within an enormously challenging policymaking environment.

But whatever the political constraints, CLASS also demonstrates that eventually design matters, too. As Eric Patashnik has noted, "what is required to *initiate* policy reform should not be confused with what is required to *sustain* it." He emphasizes that there are two distinct and important phases to the policy reform process. The first phase entails the process of shepherding a reform idea from conception through to adoption as law. This phase "is a puzzle that requires a *political* explanation." The second phase "begins the moment *after* the curtain falls on the high drama of legislative enactments." It is at this point "that reform ideas meet the tough realities of democratic politics. All the political compromises and administrative complexities that were denied or papered over during the adoption phase will show themselves, sooner if not later."[15] In the case of CLASS, it was sooner.

The fundamental problem with CLASS was that once one got beyond all the smoke and mirrors, three key provisions of the doomed program remained: no one was required to participate; almost everyone—including those with the greatest needs—would be allowed to enroll; and it had to be to be financially self-sustaining. Unfortunately, these provisions work at cross-purposes. The insurance-based model, be it private or public, requires at least one of the following: mandatory participation, underwriting, or subsidies. CLASS had none of these.

Bearing the CLASS experience in mind, it is worth considering other paths to reforming America's long-term care system. Unfortunately, and as the CLASS advocates knew all too well, they all have significant drawbacks in terms of adequacy or political feasibility. One common feature that limits their potential is the lack of awareness and understanding of the long-term care challenge on the part of the American public.

A key distinction between the various approaches to reform is whether participation should be optional or mandatory. From a strictly policy perspective, a mandatory program would be the easiest and most elegant approach. A mandatory program could be predicated on private insurance, like the Affordable Care Act, or on the social insurance model, like Medicare. The kind of coverage mandated—ranging from minimal catastrophic coverage to maximum comprehensive coverage—would be open to debate.

It is instructive to note that long-term care is far from a uniquely American problem and that other countries have already addressed it. Indeed, all wealthy, industrialized nations are facing similar concerns as the United States and for the same reason: aging populations. These other similarly situated countries have typically approached long-term care through the social insurance model. To take just one example, Germany instituted its social insurance program in 1995 largely to relieve local governments, which were bearing the burden of increased nursing home usage. The German program is funded by a mandatory 1.95 percent payroll tax split evenly between employers and employees, and individuals can choose between carrying the public plan or purchasing comparable private coverage. While the program has proven more costly than initially thought (and one estimate suggests the tax rate will need to be increased to 3.2 percent by 2040), it has been a real success in reducing the number of people relying on means-tested public programs and in easing the burden on local governments.[16] American states would, of course, be delighted to receive similar relief from their Medicaid obligations. Examples from abroad provide plenty of opportunities for policy learning that could be useful in thinking through reform ideas here.

Returning to this side of the Atlantic, and momentarily putting aside the political plausibility of a mandate, a sensible plan designed to address the largest concerns facing individuals, families, and American society would look to reduce the risk of catastrophic expenses that lead to impoverishment for the middle class and to ease the burden on Medicaid (and thereby the states). Such a plan should probably be limited to the elderly for several reasons (though reforms targeted to younger individuals with disabilities could be undertaken separately). First, it is the aging of the American population that poses the great challenge to the nation. Second, disabilities incurred by the non-elderly are often difficult to anticipate, whereas we know that there is a strong chance that people living to the age of sixty-five will encounter challenges related to aging; these needs are easy to anticipate and it is reasonable to expect people to make provisions for this likelihood. Third, the two groups typically have different goals and needs. Younger individuals with disabilities often want to work, and they frequently have family situations that are different from those over the age of sixty-five.

The basic outlines of such a plan would be relatively straightforward. A requirement to carry private, government-approved catastrophic long-term care coverage would be oriented toward addressing nursing home care because that is where the burden and risk is greatest for the middle class and state governments. Like the Affordable Care Act does for health insurance, subsidies would need to be provided for low-income earners. The coverage might resemble plans that are already available on the private market. Because the average nursing home stay is about three years, individuals could be required to carry a plan covering that length of time. A more costly approach might require coverage spanning five or six years, a period that encompasses the vast majority of nursing home stays. The benefit level could be indexed to nursing home costs, though, like CLASS, it could be disbursed in the form of a cash payment that would permit individuals more flexibility and allow for noninstitutional care when feasible. As noted in chapter 1, the average cost of a bed in a shared room is about $81,000 per year, which could be covered entirely with a daily benefit of about $220. Individuals living beyond the covered years might immediately become eligible for Medicaid coverage. Such a provision would maintain Medicaid's role in long-term care, but greatly reduce costs because far fewer people would be relying on the program for coverage. If everyone was required to participate, something along these general lines would be entirely feasible at an affordable premium level.

Of course, as the CLASS advocates recognized, passing a program with mandatory participation is far more difficult politically. In the late 1980s and early 1990s, the idea of an individual mandate for health insurance was developed at the conservative Heritage Foundation and garnered support from leading Republicans such as Speaker of the House Newt Gingrich and Senate Majority Leader Bob Dole, who saw it as an alternative to the Clinton administration's approach to health reform. The individual mandate later came to form the basis of Republican Governor Mitt

Romney's overhaul of the Massachusetts health-care system.[17] But now, after the acrimony over the Affordable Care Act's individual mandate for health insurance, this route appears even more daunting for long-term care. Nonetheless, the case for mandated long-term care insurance coverage is actually stronger than it was for general health insurance. The premise of the individual mandate for health insurance was that it was necessary to prevent healthy people from gaming a system in which insurers were required to cover all applicants regardless of preexisting conditions. Policymakers (and insurance companies) argued that if insurers were going to be required to cover anyone who applied, there had to also be a requirement that everyone carry insurance. Otherwise, the system would incentivize healthy people to go without coverage until they were sick or injured. Insurers would then be in the untenable position of covering those needing care without a pool of healthy people paying into the system. That logic applies even more to long-term care coverage, where the problem is not confined to a cost-benefit analysis on the part of consumers, but also involves high degrees of ignorance and confusion—issues that are far less of a problem for standard health insurance.

Other fiscal and political concerns associated with the history of entitlements also argue against a mandatory program. Over time, entitlement programs like Medicare and Social Security have cost more than initially projected and faced considerable pressure to increase and expand benefits.[18] It is not unwarranted, then, to worry that creating a new long-term care entitlement would yield more of the same in this regard. More broadly, some would certainly object on the grounds that adding a long-term care entitlement would be another step toward the kind of "nanny state" that Alexis de Tocqueville, among others, has cautioned is bad for the soul of the democratic citizen and, ultimately, for the fate of liberal democracy itself. Cradle-to-grave dependence on a benevolent government—as memorably depicted in President Obama's 2012 "Life of Julia" campaign ad—may sound reassuring, the argument goes, but it risks sapping the vitality and dynamism that allow individuals and societies to flourish. Yet even if one is sympathetic to this general critique, it is far from clear that long-term care is the best ground on which to contest this principle. Nonetheless, it is an effective, if somewhat crude and undiscerning, argument that would be leveled against any proposed new entitlement, worthy or not.

In contrast to the mandatory model, a voluntary approach greatly reduces the political hurdles. The basic idea here would be to create new incentives for individuals to provide for their own security by purchasing private long-term care coverage. Experiments with this approach have already been undertaken. The federal government and dozens of states offer varying types of tax incentives for individuals who purchase private insurance. One optional program allows purchasers of long-term care coverage to qualify for Medicaid immediately after their private benefits expire, thereby allowing individuals to avoid impoverishment and promising to bring relief to government budgets by decreasing reliance on Medicaid. To date, however, these initiatives have had only marginal success in increasing participation and have failed to significantly reduce state Medicaid expenditures.[19]

Advocates of this general approach maintain that part of the reason why initial efforts have had underwhelming results is due to the unintentionally distorting role of Medicaid. Stephen Moses of the Center for Long-Term Care Reform, for instance, argues that "[i]n America today, you can ignore the risk of long-term care, avoid the premiums for private insurance, wait to see if you ever become chronically ill, and if you do need expensive long-term care someday, the government will pay for it" through Medicaid.[20] As a result, adherents of this approach claim that Medicaid should be reformed to make it less appealing as a long-term care financing option. Doing so would presumably incentivize individuals to purchase private plans.

Theoretically, boosting private insurance would help address the long-term care problem, but the ignorance and confusion that characterize this policy area are formidable barriers. Limiting the appeal of Medicaid to incentivize private coverage, for instance, assumes a degree of knowledge and rationalization on the part of the American public that is not currently in evidence. Most individuals are not making a calculated decision to forgo private insurance because they know they can freeload off Medicaid.

Given the lack of interest in private insurance and general misunderstanding, it is not clear how creating new incentives would significantly counter the projected spike in demand accompanying the aging of the baby boomers. Thus, the clear downside to the nonmandatory approach is that, whatever marginal advantages it may hold, there is little reason to think that reforms in this vein would do much to address the larger problem of America's dysfunctional long-term care system or bring much relief to state governments.

If any hope exists of shaking up the status quo on the subject of long-term care, it will require a concerted campaign of public education to raise awareness of the challenges the current system poses for individuals, families, and American society. At some point, it will be impossible to ignore, but government budgets—not to mention many individuals and families—would benefit greatly by taking action before the full-fledged crisis hits. Greater awareness would improve the chances for all reform possibilities. For the idea of mandating coverage, increased awareness might reduce the political hurdles. The Affordable Care Act experience currently makes it difficult to envision a point at which a long-term care mandate would be politically viable, though the situation might change if the Obama health reform comes to be seen as a success and is more widely embraced. Increased awareness would also be a boon to any effort predicated on increasing the number of people choosing to carry private coverage.

Opening a 2007 hearing on CLASS before the Senate HELP Committee, Ted Kennedy identified long-term care as "one of the most pressing and personal issues our Nation will face.... The issue is about all of us. I was here, in the U.S. Senate, when we passed the Medicare program.... But what we never really anticipated is the kind of situation that we're [facing] today [in which] countless senior citizens and persons with disabilities still live in poverty.... That was never the intent of the public assistance programs." The CLASS Act was Kennedy's response to this problem, one he hoped would empower individuals and families while also reducing "the mushrooming costs of Medicaid."[21] As it turned out, CLASS was unable to meet those lofty ambitions. However, there is no doubt that Kennedy's diagnosis of the problem was on the mark.

In the months following the Obama administration's decision to drop CLASS, the policy's advocates, channeling their late champion, launched a national effort to pressure political leaders to either revive their fallen program or identify a viable alternative. Their standard refrain was "If not CLASS, then what?" This question has not been answered, but it cannot be ignored indefinitely.

State Spending by Function as a Percent of Total State Expenditures, 2010

	Elem. & secondary education	Higher education	Public assistance	Medicaid	Corrections	Trans-portation	All other
Alabama	24.3%	21.4%	0.2%	25.8%	2.9%	8.2%	17.1%
Alaska	14.6	8.6	1.2	12.0	3.2	17.0	43.4
Arizona	22.0	12.6	0.3	27.7	3.8	5.6	28.0
Arkansas	17.2	15.3	2.2	20.0	2.1	4.9	38.2
California	19.6	8.1	4.9	18.9	3.9	5.3	39.2
Colorado	24.7	14.2	0.0	15.3	2.6	4.6	38.6
Connecticut	20.1	13.9	2.5	25.4	3.4	9.5	25.2
Delaware	23.8	4.2	0.5	14.4	2.9	8.6	45.5
Florida	20.5	7.7	0.3	30.0	4.8	9.4	27.2
Georgia	24.6	17.1	1.4	19.5	3.0	6.2	28.3
Hawaii	15.6	8.8	0.8	13.3	2.0	9.7	49.7
Idaho	27.4	7.7	0.3	23.0	3.3	10.4	27.9
Illinois	18.2	4.5	0.2	23.6	2.0	8.1	43.3
Indiana	32.4	7.1	1.4	23.1	2.9	10.6	22.4
Iowa	17.3	24.4	0.7	18.6	2.4	9.1	27.5
Kansas	25.5	16.1	0.4	18.8	2.6	8.3	28.3
Kentucky	19.4	22.4	0.8	21.9	2.2	8.0	25.2
Louisiana	18.1	8.0	0.6	23.7	2.9	10.9	35.7
Maine	17.6	3.3	2.6	28.6	2.0	7.8	38.1
Maryland	21.0	14.4	3.1	20.4	4.7	4.6	31.8
Massachusetts	12.9	7.9	2.5	18.8	2.5	6.9	48.6
Michigan	28.4	4.5	1.1	24.2	4.7	7.4	29.7
Minnesota	21.7	10.7	1.5	25.1	1.6	9.8	29.6

	Elem. & secondary education	Higher education	Public assistance	Medicaid	Corrections	Transportation	All other
Mississippi	17.1	15.3	0.2	22.9	1.8	7.3	35.4
Missouri	21.3	5.2	0.7	34.4	2.7	11.2	24.6
Montana	15.1	9.6	0.6	15.4	3.0	11.5	44.8
Nebraska	15.7	22.4	0.6	17.2	2.3	7.4	34.4
Nevada	21.5	10.8	0.7	18.3	3.9	11.4	33.5
N. Hampshire	19.0	5.0	1.8	24.9	1.9	9.2	38.1
New Jersey	24.6	7.9	0.9	21.3	3.5	9.9	32.0
New Mexico	21.1	18.0	1.1	22.1	1.9	8.8	27.0
New York	20.4	7.5	3.0	28.7	2.7	6.1	31.5
No. Carolina	19.3	12.4	0.5	24.2	2.9	7.1	33.5
North Dakota	16.6	20.7	0.2	13.7	1.8	11.3	35.8
Ohio	20.2	4.9	1.8	21.3	3.4	4.9	43.5
Oklahoma	13.5	19.5	1.0	17.1	2.4	7.2	39.3
Oregon	11.6	7.1	0.4	13.1	3.0	5.6	59.2
Pennsylvania	19.8	3.3	2.2	29.6	3.4	10.1	31.6
Rhode Island	14.1	11.8	1.5	25.0	2.2	5.3	40.1
So. Carolina	17.1	20.9	0.3	22.6	2.8	9.1	27.0
South Dakota	15.4	17.3	0.8	21.7	2.8	13.7	28.5
Tennessee	17.7	13.1	0.5	28.8	2.3	6.4	31.3
Texas	29.3	10.0	0.3	24.6	4.0	7.2	24.6
Utah	18.9	9.5	0.9	11.9	2.6	25.9	30.4
Vermont	33.0	2.2	2.2	25.9	2.9	9.8	23.8
Virginia	16.7	15.6	0.5	16.1	3.2	9.2	38.7
Washington	24.4	13.2	1.4	23.0	3.2	9.1	25.8
West Virginia	10.6	11.9	0.6	12.6	1.1	5.8	57.4
Wisconsin	18.1	12.3	0.3	17.1	3.1	7.1	41.9
Wyoming	11.7	5.3	0.0	7.3	1.6	13.2	61.0
All States	20.5%	10.2%	1.6%	22.3%	3.1%	7.7%	34.6%

SOURCE: National Association of State Budget Officers, *State Expenditure Report 2010* (2011), Table 5, 11.

CHAPTER 1

1. Kathleen Sebelius, "The CLASS Program," *Huffington Post*, October 14, 2011, http://www.huffingtonpost.com/sec-kathleen-sebelius/the-class-program_b_1011270.html.

2. Ezra Klein, "What the CLASS Act Says about Health-Care Reform," *Washington Post*, October 17, 2011, http://www.washingtonpost.com/blogs/wonkblog/post/what-the-class-act-says-about-health-care-reform/2011/08/25/gIQA8cL0rL_blog.html; Kevin Drum, "The CLASS Act and Good Government," *Mother Jones*, October 15, 2011, http://www.motherjones.com/kevin-drum/2011/10/class-act-and-good-government; Jonathan Cohn, "A Setback for Obamacare? Or Vindication? How about Both," *The New Republic*, October 17, 2011, http://www.newrepublic.com/blog/jonathan-cohn/96332/class-act-obamacare-long-term-care-mandate-cost-foster.

3. Kent Conrad of North Dakota made this charge. Lori Montgomery, "Proposed Long-Term Insurance Program Raises Questions," *Washington Post*, October 27, 2009, http://articles.washingtonpost.com/2009-10-27/politics/36874585_1_larry-minnix-long-term-care-insurance-program.

4. Douglas W. Elmendorf, letter to Harry Reid, November 18, 2009, http://www.cbo.gov/sites/default/files/cbofiles/ftpdocs/107xx/doc10731/reid_letter_11_18_09.pdf.

5. Sebelius, "The CLASS Program."

6. Interview with Republican congressional staffer, February 24, 2012.

7. Judith Feder, "The Missing Piece: Medicare, Medicaid, and Long-Term Care," in *Medicare and Medicaid at 50: America's Entitlement Programs in the Age of Affordable Care*, edited by Alan B. Cohen, David C. Colby, Keith A. Wailoo, and Julian E. Zelizer (New York: Oxford University Press, 2015), 264.

8. Peter Kemper, Harriet L. Komisar, and Lisa Alecxih, "Long-Term Care Over an Uncertain Future: What Can Current Retirees Expect?" *Inquiry* 42.4 (Winter 2005–2006), 335–350; Susan Rogers and Harriet L. Komisar, "Who Needs Long-Term Care?" Georgetown University Long-Term Care Financing Project. 2003, http://hpi.georgetown.edu/ltc/papers.html.

9. H. Stephen Kaye, Charlene Harrington, and Mitchell P. LaPlante, "Long-Term Care: Who Gets It, Who Provides It, Who Pays, and How Much?" *Health Affairs*

29.1 (2010):11–21; U.S. Department of Health and Human Services and U.S. Department of Labor, "The Future Supply of Long-Term Care Workers in Relation to the Aging Baby Boom Generation," Report to Congress, May 14, 2003, http:// aspe.hhs.gov/daltcp/reports/ltcwork.htm#note1; Susan Rogers and Harriet L. Komisar, "Who Needs Long-Term Care?"; Kemper, Komisar, and Alecxih, "Long-Term Care Over an Uncertain Future: What Can Current Retirees Expect?" *Inquiry* 42.4 (Winter 2005–2006): 335–350.

10. Sandra R. Levitsky, *Caring for Our Own: Why There Is No Political Demand for New American Social Welfare Rights* (New York: Oxford University Press, 2014).

11. Carol V. O'Shaughnessy, "National Spending for Long-Term Services and Supports (LTSS), 2012," *National Health Policy Forum*, March 27, 2014, http://www.nhpf. org/library/the-basics/Basics_LTSS_03-27-14.pdf; Nicholas Barr, "Long-Term Care: A Suitable Case for Social Insurance," *Social Policy and Administration* 44.4 (2010): 359–374; Lynn Feinberg, Susan C. Reinhard, Ari Houser, and Rita Choula, "Valuing the Invaluable: 2011 Update; The Economic Value of Family Caregiving in 2009," *Insight on the Issues*, AARP Public Policy Institute 51 (2011), http://assets. aarp.org/rgcenter/ppi/ltc/i51-caregiving.pdf; Kaye, Harrington, and LaPlante, "Long-Term Care: Who Gets It, Who Provides It, Who Pays, and How Much?" 19.

12. Some overviews of long-term care spending include Medicare as a payer. In these assessments, Medicaid's portion of overall spending appears lower, usually around half. Other overviews exclude Medicare from considerations of long-term care spending because that program covers only acute and post-acute medical care for seniors. Medicare will cover only 100 days of institution-based care that is oriented toward rehabilitating patients. Long-term care (i.e., care without the expectation of rehabilitation) is not part of Medicare's mission. O'Shaughnessy, "National Spending for Long-Term Services and Supports (LTSS), 2012," 3.

13. National Conference for State Legislatures, "Top Fiscal Issues for 2014 Legislative Sessions," December 30, 2013, http://www.ncsl.org/research/fiscal-policy/top-fiscal-issues-for-2014-legislative-sessions.aspx; National Conference for State Legislatures, "Top Fiscal Issues for 2013 Legislative Sessions," January 3, 2013, http://www.ncsl.org/research/fiscal-policy/top-fiscal-issues-for-2013-legislative-sessions.aspx.

14. U.S. Department of Health and Human Services, "Paying for LTC," 2012; U.S. Department of Health and Human Services and U.S. Department of Labor, "The Future Supply of Long-Term Care Workers in Relation to the Aging Baby Boom Generation."

15. The same is true for disabled individuals of working age. See Andrea Louise Campbell, *Trapped in America's Safety Net: One Family's Struggle* (Chicago: University of Chicago Press, 2014).

16. Kaiser Commission on Medicaid Facts, "Medicaid and Long-Term Care Services and Supports," 2009, http://kaiserfamilyfoundation.files.wordpress.com/2013/01/2186-09.pdf.

17. U.S. Department of Health and Human Services, "Paying for LTC," 2012, O'Shaughnessy, "National Spending for Long-Term Services and Supports (LTSS), 2012"; Barr, "Long-Term Care: A Suitable Case for Social Insurance."

18. Jeffrey R. Brown and Amy Finkelstein, "Insuring Long-Term Care in the United States," *Journal of Economic Perspectives* 25.4 (Fall 2011): 129.

19. "Long-Term Care in America: Expectations and Reality," Associated Press-NORC Center for Public Affairs Research, May 2014, http://www.longtermcarepoll. org/PDFs/LTC%202014/AP-NORC-Long-Term%20Care%20in%20America_ FINAL%20WEB.pdf.

20. For an extensive and broader discussion of the obstacles in challenging America's "taken-for-granted assumptions about social welfare provision" (167), see Levitsky, *Caring for Our Own*, especially chapter 7.

21. Edward Kennedy, Tom Harkin, John Dingell, and Frank Pallone, "Kennedy, Harkin, Dingell, Pallone Introduce CLASS ACT: New Bipartisan Insurance Program Would Help Those with Severe Functional Impairments Gain Independence," Press Release, July 10, 2007.

22. Kennedy, Harkin, Dingell, and Pallone, "Kennedy, Harkin, Dingell, Pallone Introduce CLASS ACT"; Kaiser Family Foundation, "The Sleeper in Health Reform: Long-Term Care and the CLASS Act," October 20, 2009, http://kaiserfamilyfoundation.files.wordpress.com/2013/01/102009_kff_class_act_transcript_final.pdf; Patient Protection and Affordable Care Act, Public Law 111–148 (2010), 828.

24. Interview with former CBO staffer, February 23, 2012.

25. Vesting periods are also common in other areas, particularly in pension plans. When it was initially implemented, Social Security also had a prefunding period. The first payroll taxes were collected in 1937, but benefits did not begin until 1940.

26. Douglas W. Elmendorf, letter to Kay R. Hagan, July 6, 2009, http://www.cbo.gov/ ftpdocs/104xx/doc10436/07-06-CLASSAct.pdf.

27. Interview with Republican congressional staffer, February 24, 2012.

28. Barack Obama, "Remarks by the President after Meeting with Senate Democrats," The White House, December 15, 2009, http://www.whitehouse.gov/the-press-office/remarks-president-after-meeting-with-senate-democrats.

29. Karl W. Deutsch, *The Nerves of Government* (New York: The Free Press, 1966); Peter Hall, "Policy Paradigms, Social Learning and the State: The Case of Economic Policy Making in Britain," *Comparative Politics* 25.3 (1993): 275–296; Mark Peterson, "The Limits of Social Learning: Translating Analysis into Action," *Journal of Health Politics, Policy, and Law* 22.4 (1997): 1078–1114; Margaret Weir and Theda Skocpol, "State Structures and the Possibilities for 'Keynesian' Responses to the Great Depression in Sweden, Britain, and the United States," in *Bringing the State Back In*, edited by Peter B. Evans, Dietrich Rueschemeyer, and Theda Skocpol (New York: Cambridge University Press, 1985), 107–167; Richard Rose, *Lesson-Drawing in Public Policy* (Chatham, NJ: Chatham House, 1993); Hugh Heclo, *Modern Social Politics in Britain and Sweden* (New Haven, CT: Yale University Press, 1974).

30. Peterson, "The Limits of Social Learning," 1080.

31. Peter J. May, "Policy Learning and Failure," *Journal of Public Policy* 12.4 (1992): 340.

32. Peter J. May, "Politics and Policy Analysis," *Political Science Quarterly* 101.1 (1986): 109–125; Paul A. Sabatier, "An Advocacy Coalition Framework of Policy

Change and the Role of Policy-Oriented Learning Therein," *Policy Sciences* 21 (1988): 129–168.

33. Campbell, *How Policies Make Citizens: Senior Political Activism and the Welfare State* (Princeton, NJ: Princeton University Press, 2005); Paul Pierson, "Policy Feedbacks and Political Change: Contrasting Reagan and Thatcher's Pension-Reform Initiatives," *Studies in American Political Development* 6 (1992): 359–390; Theda Skocpol, *Protecting Soldiers and Mothers: The Political Origins of Social Policy in the United States* (Cambridge, MA: Harvard University Press, 1992).

34. Thomas A. Birkland, *Lessons of Disaster: Policy Change after Catastrophic Events* (Washington, DC: Georgetown University Press, 2006); May, "Policy Learning and Failure."

35. While the lessons drawn from history are often influential, they may or may not be entirely accurate. Jacob S. Hacker notes that many of the "putative lessons" drawn from complex political events "turn out to be hastily formulated, weakly grounded and prescriptively inadequate." Hacker, "Learning from Defeat? Political Analysis and the Failure of Health Care Reform in the United States," *British Journal of Political Science* 31 (2001): 61.

36. Richard E. Neustadt and Harvey V. Fineberg, *The Swine Flu Affair: Decision-Making on a Slippery Disease* (Washington, DC: U.S. Department of Health, Education, and Welfare, 1978); Jeffrey L. Pressman and Aaron Wildavsky, *Implementation* (Berkeley: University of California Press, 1973); Sven Steinmo and Jon Watts, "It's the Institutions, Stupid! Why Comprehensive National Health Insurance Always Fails in America," *Journal of Health Politics, Policy and Law* 20.2 (1995): 329–372.

37. This approach to conducting interviews is common in political science and health policy research. See, for example, Frank R. Baumgartner, Jeffrey M. Berry, Marie Hojnacki, David C. Kimball, and Beth L. Leech, *Lobbying and Policy Change: Who Wins, Who Loses, and Why* (Chicago: University of Chicago Press, 2009), 272–273; John E. McDonough, *Inside National Health Reform* (Berkeley: University of California Press, 2011), 8–9; Neustadt and Fineberg, *The Swine Flu Affair*; Joshua M. Wiener, Carroll L. Estes, Susan M. Goldenson, and Sheryl C. Goldberg, "What Happened to Long-Term Care in the Health Reform Debate of 1993–1994? Lessons for the Future," *The Milbank Quarterly* 79.2 (2001): 208. Most interviews were conducted in 2012. Most were done in-person in Washington, DC, though some took place in various other locations or by phone.

CHAPTER 2

1. James Madison, "Federalist 58," *The Federalist Papers*, 1788.

2. Harold D. Lasswell, *Politics: Who Gets What, When, How* (New York: Whittlesey House, 1936).

3. A substantial body of work is available analyzing the contemporary policymaking process. For an overview of the contemporary legislative process, see James M. Curry, *Legislating in the Dark* (Chicago: University of Chicago Press, 2015); Barbara Sinclair, *Unorthodox Lawmaking: New Legislative Processes in the U.S. Congress* (Washington, DC: Congressional Quarterly Press, 1997). On the rise

of omnibus legislation, see Diana Evans, *Greasing the Wheels: The Use of Pork Barrel Projects to Build Majority Coalitions in Congress* (New York: Cambridge University Press, 2004); Glen Krutz, *Hitching a Ride: Omnibus Legislating in the U.S. Congress* (Columbus: Ohio State University Press, 2001). On the Budget Act of 1974 and its effects, see Louis Fisher, "Presidential Budgetary Duties," *Presidential Studies Quarterly* 42.4 (2012): 754–790; James A. Thurber, "Centralization, Devolution, and Turf Protection in the Congressional Budget Process," in *Congress Reconsidered*, 6th ed., edited by Lawrence C. Dodd and Bruce I. Oppenheimer (Washington, DC: Congressional Quarterly Press, 1997), 325–346; James A. Thurber, "The Dynamics and Dysfunction of the Congressional Budget Process: From Inception to Deadlock," in *Congress Reconsidered*, 10th ed., edited by Lawrence C. Dodd and Bruce I. Oppenheimer (Washington, DC: Congressional Quarterly Press, 2013), 319–346. On the Congressional Budget Office, see Philip G. Joyce, *The Congressional Budget Office: Honest Numbers, Power, and Policymaking* (Washington, DC: Georgetown University Press, 2011).

4. Richard F. FennoJr., *Congressmen in Committees* (Boston: Little, Brown, 1973).

5. See, for instance: Jesse Burkhead, *Government Budgeting* (New York: John Wiley & Sons, 1956); Arthur Smithies, *The Budgetary Process in the United States* (New York: McGraw-Hill, 1955). For a foundational, normative exploration of how budgeting ought to work that animated calls for reform, see: V. O. KeyJr., "The Lack of a Budgetary Theory," *American Political Science Review* 34.6 (1940): 1137–1144.

6. Julian E. Zelizer, *On Capitol Hill: The Struggle to Reform Congress and Its Consequences, 1948–2000* (New York: Cambridge University Press, 2004), 152. From 1931 to 1957, Southern Democrats chaired Ways and Means for all but two Congresses in which Republicans held the majority; Wilbur Mills (AR) was then chairman from 1958 to 1974. A similar pattern played out on House Appropriations where George Mahon (TX) held the gavel from 1964 to 1979. Southern Democrats also presided over Senate Finance from 1933 to 1981, except for a pair of two year stints under GOP control. Finally, Southern Democrats chaired Senate Appropriations from 1969 to 1977.

7. Office of Management and Budget, "Table 1.1—Summary of Receipts, Outlays, and Surpluses or Deficits (-): 1789–2019" and "Table 1.3—Summary of Receipts, Outlays, and Surpluses or Deficits (-) in Current Dollars, Constant (FY 2009) Dollars, and as Percentage of GDP: 1940–2019," http://www.whitehouse.gov/omb/budget/Historicals.

8. John W. Ellwood and James A. Thurber, "The Politics of the Congressional Budget Process Re-examined," in *Congress Reconsidered*, 2nd ed., edited by Lawrence C. Dodd and Bruce I. Oppenheimer (Washington, DC: Congressional Quarterly Press, 1981), 247–251.

9. David R. Mayhew, *Congress: The Electoral Connection* (New Haven, CT: Yale University Press, 1974), 149–158.

10. Mayhew, *Congress*, 155; Randall Strahan, *New Ways and Means: Reform and Change in a Congressional Committee* (Chapel Hill: University of North Carolina Press, 1990), 12; John Manley, *The Politics of Finance: The House Committee on Ways and*

Means (Boston: Little, Brown, 1970), 21–22, 63–90, 110; Fenno, *Congressmen in Committees*, 83–86.

11. Aaron Wildavsky, *The Politics of the Budgetary Process* (Boston: Little, Brown, 1964), 47; Richard F. FennoJr., *The Power of the Purse: Appropriations Politics in Congress* (Boston: Little, Brown, 1966), 98–102.

12. Fenno, *Congressmen in Committees*, 88.

13. Manley, *The Politics of Finance*, 72–73.

14. Strahan, *New Ways and Means*, 13–14; Manley, *The Politics of Finance*, 111.

15. Fenno, *Congressmen in Committees*, 86.

16. Strahan, *New Ways and Means*, 12; Manley, *The Politics of Finance*, 268–291; Fenno, *Congressmen in Committees*, 153–154.

17. Martha Derthick, *Policymaking for Social Security* (Washington, DC: Brookings Institution Press, 1979), 49; Manley, *The Politics of Finance*, 281; Allen Schick, *Congress and Money: Budgeting, Spending and Taxing* (New York: Urban Institute, 1980), chapter 12.

18. Mayhew, *Congress*, 154, 158; Julian E. Zelizer, *Taxing America: Wilbur D. Mills, Congress, and the State, 1945–1975* (New York: Cambridge University Press, 1998), 42.

19. Wildavsky, *How to Limit Government Spending* (Berkeley: University of California Press, 1980), 56; Wildavsky, *The Politics of the Budgetary Process*.

20. Wildavsky, *The Politics of the Budgetary Process*, 178, 131–132.

21. Lyndon Baines Johnson, *The Vantage Point: Perspectives on the Presidency, 1963–1969* (New York: Holt, Rinehart, and Winston, 1971), 214.

22. David Blumenthal and James A. Morone, *The Heart of Power: Health and Politics in the Oval Office* (Berkeley: University of California Press, 2010), 185–205.

23. Francis M. Bator, "No Good Choices: LBJ and the Vietnam/Great Society Connection," *Diplomatic History* 32.3 (2008): 309–340.

24. John McCormack, audiotape, 4:54 P.M., March 23, 1965, "Recordings and Transcripts of Conversations," Citation 7141, http://millercenter.org/scripps/archive/presidentialrecordings/johnson/1965/03_1965.

25. Ibid. *Alcalde* is a Spanish word for mayor or judge.

26. Ibid.

27. Ibid.

28. Edward Kennedy, audiotape, 11:32 A.M., January 9, 1965, "Recording and Transcripts of Conversations," Citation 6718, http://millercenter.org/scripps/archive/presidentialrecordings/johnson/1965/01_1965.

29. Even when controlling for inflation, spending had nearly doubled over this period. Office of Management and Budget, "Table 1.1" and "Table 1.3."

30. Strahan, *New Ways and Means*, 25.

31. Eric M. Patashnik, "Congress and the Budget since 1974," in *The American Congress: The Building of Democracy*, edited by Julian E. Zelizer, (New York: Houghton Mifflin, 2004), 671. The Vietnam War was a further drain on government coffers. American combat forces hit the ground in Southeast Asia just five months before President Johnson signed the bill creating Medicare and Medicaid. However, defense spending declined as a percentage of total spending. In 1962, it represented

49 percent of federal spending; in 1968, 46 percent; in 1971, 37.5 percent; and in 1974, 29.5 percent. Nooree Lee, "Congressional Budget and Impoundment Control Act of 1974, Reconsidered," Harvard Law School Federal Budget Policy Seminar, Briefing Paper No. 34, April 29, 2008, 7.

32. Allen Schick, *Congress and Money: Budgeting, Spending and Taxing* (New York: Urban Institute, 1980), 26.

33. Two points of clarification: (1) Mandatory spending is not synonymous with entitlement programs. In addition to entitlements, mandatory spending encompasses an array of smaller outlays such as pay for members of Congress and interest payments on the national debt. But entitlement programs account for the vast majority of mandatory spending. (2) Entitlements include, but are by no means limited to, Social Security, Medicare, and Medicaid. Other entitlement programs include unemployment insurance and the Supplemental Nutritional Assistance Program (formerly known as Food Stamps). Compared to the big three entitlements, these other programs require much smaller commitments from federal coffers. In terms of overall mandatory spending, Social Security accounts for approximately 38 percent, Medicare 27 percent, and Medicaid 12 percent. In terms of overall spending (i.e., mandatory and discretionary outlays), Social Security accounts for 22 percent, Medicare 16 percent, and Medicaid 7 percent. Source: Congressional Budget Office, "Historical Budget Data—February 2013," http://cbo.gov/publication/43904.

34. Congressional Budget Office, "Historical Budget Data"; Center for Budget and Policy Priorities, "Policy Basics: Non-defense Discretionary Programs," April 20, 2014, http://www.cbpp.org/cms/?fa=view&id=3973; Nicholas Eberstadt, *A Nation of Takers: America's Entitlement Epidemic* (West Conshohocken, PA: Templeton Press, 2012), 19.

35. The National Commission on Fiscal Responsibility of Reform, "The Moment of Truth," December 2010, https://www.fiscalcommission.gov/sites/fiscalcommission.gov/files/documents/TheMomentofTruth12_1_2010.pdf.

36. Eberstadt, *A Nation of Takers*.

37. Will Marshall, "Investments and Entitlements," *The American Prospect*, Forum on Progressive Perspectives on the Future of the New Deal/Great Society Entitlement Programs, January 29, 2014, http://prospect.org/article/investments-and-entitlements#.UumBu_ldUYG.

38. Patashnik, "Congress and the Budget since 1974," 672; Ellwood and Thurber, "The Politics of the Congressional Budget Process Re-examined," 248.

39. Patashnik, "Congress and the Budget since 1974," 671–672.

40. Ellwood and Thurber, "The Politics of the Congressional Budget Process Re-examined"; Daniel J. Palazzolo, *The Speaker and the Budget: Leadership in the Post-reform House of Representatives* (Pittsburgh: University of Pittsburgh Press, 1992), 31; Patashnik, "Congress and the Budget since 1974," 671–673.

41. Patashnik, "Congress and the Budget since 1974," 675.

42. Richard Nixon, "Special Message to the Congress on Federal Government Spending," July 26, 1972, http://www.presidency.ucsb.edu/ws/?pid=3506.

43. Schick, *Congress and Money*.

44. Ibid., 46; Patashnik, "Congress and the Budget," 673.

45. W. Thomas Wander, "The Politics of Congressional Budget Reform," in *Congressional Budgeting: Politics, Process, and Power*, edited by W. Thomas Wander, Ted Herbert, and Gary W. Copeland, (Baltimore: Johns Hopkins University Press, 1984), 9.

46. Patashnik, "Congress and the Budget since 1974," 674.

47. Joyce, *The Congressional Budget Office*, 21–22.

48. Congressional Budget Office, "An Introduction to the Congressional Budget Office," November 2014, https://www.cbo.gov/sites/default/files/cbofiles/attachments/2014-IntroToCBO-2.pdf.

49. Sinclair, *Unorthodox Lawmaking*.

50. Richard Nixon, "Remarks on Signing the Congressional Budget and Impoundment Control Act of 1974," July 12, 1974, http://www.presidency.ucsb.edu/ws/?pid=4293; Nixon, "Statement about the Congressional Budget and Impoundment Control Act of 1974," July 12, 1974, http://www.presidency.ucsb.edu/ws/?pid=4294.

51. Fisher, "Ten Years of the Budget Act: Still Searching for Controls," *Public Budgeting and Finance* (Autumn 1985): 3.

52. The Budget Act was followed by a long string of failed budget fixes like Gramm-Rudman-Hollings and the Joint Select Committee on Deficit Reduction.

53. Fisher, "Federal Budget Doldrums: The Vacuum in Presidential Leadership," *Public Administration Review* 50.6 (1990): 693.

54. James A. Thurber, "The Dynamics and Dysfunction of the Congressional Budget Process: From Inception to Deadlock," in *Congress Reconsidered*, 10th ed., edited by Lawrence C. Dodd and Bruce I. Oppenheimer (Washington, DC: CQ Press, 2013), 334–336.

55. See, for example, Fisher, "Ten Years of the Budget Act."

56. U.S. Congress, House Committee on Rules, "Congressional Budget Process," hearings, pt. 1, 97th Cong., 2nd Sess. (1982), 239.

57. Statement by Rudolph Penner, U.S. Congress, House Committee on the Budget, "Budget Process Reform," hearings, 101st Cong., 2nd Sess. (1990), 20–21.

58. Joyce, *The Congressional Budget Office*. See also: Thurber, "The Dynamics and Dysfunction of the Congressional Budget Process," 336.

59. Donald B. Marron, "Understanding CBO Health Cost Estimates," The Heritage Foundation, July 15, 2009, http://www.heritage.org/research/reports/2009/07/understanding-cbo-health-cost-estimates.

60. The Statutory Pay-As-You-Go Act, Public Law 111–139 (2010).

61. Joyce, *The Congressional Budget Office*, 6–7 and 224.

62. Other reforms include the 1985 Balanced Budget and Emergency Deficit Control Act (or Gramm-Rudman-Hollings I), the 1987 Balanced Budget and Emergency Deficit Control Reaffirmation Act (or Gramm-Rudman-Hollings II), the 1990 Omnibus Budget Reconciliation Act, the 1990 Budget Enforcement Act, and a 1996 amendment to Title X of the Budget Act that provided the president with the line-item veto.

63. Bill Heniff Jr., "The Budget Reconciliation Process: The Senate's 'Byrd Rule,'" Congressional Research Service, September 13, 2010, http://www.senate.gov/CRSReports/crs-publish.cfm?pid=%26*2%3C4RL_%3F%0A.

64. Aaron Wildavsky, *The Politics of the Budgetary Process*, 3rd ed. (Boston: Little, Brown, 1979), 261.

CHAPTER 3

1. Other, less prominent proposals were made during this period, too. Senator George Mitchell (D-ME), Representative Pete Stark (D-CA), and Representative Henry Waxman (D-CA) sponsored several comprehensive long-term care bills, but they were widely seen as too expensive and never got voted out of committee.

2. For a comprehensive and outstanding overview of the first fifty years of Medicare and Medicaid and how these programs have evolved from 1965 through today, see Alan B. Cohen, David C. Colby, Keith A. Wailoo, and Julian E. Zelizer, eds., *Medicare and Medicaid at 50: America's Entitlement Programs in the Age of Affordable Care* (New York: Oxford University Press, 2015).

3. U.S. Congress, Senate, *Congressional Record*, 89th Cong., 1st Sess., July 7, 1965, 15790–15809.

4. U.S. Congress, House, *Congressional Record*, 89th Cong., 1st Sess., April 7, 1965, 7201–7245.

5. See, for example: Eve Edstrom, "Long Fight to Assure Economic Security in Old Age Near Goal," *Washington Post*, April 6, 1965, A5; *Wall Street Journal*, "Benefits in House's 'Medicare' Bill Leave Little Senate Could Add, Democrats Feel," March 25, 1965, 17; *Chicago Tribune*, "Medicare Bill Benefits Seen as a Delusion," March 6, 1965, N4; Thomas J. Foley, "Medicare Change Aimed at Catastrophic Illness," *Los Angeles Times*, April 10, 1965, 4.

6. Arlen J. Large, "Medicare Mechanics," *Wall Street Journal*, March 2, 1965, 1.

7. U.S. Congress, Senate, *Congressional Record*, July 7, 1965, 15795.

8. U.S. Congress, House, *Congressional Record*, April 7, 1965, 7207.

9. For a social and intellectual history of American medicine that addresses this topic at numerous points, see Paul Starr, *The Social Transformation of American Medicine* (New York: Basic Books, 1982). On the idea of progress generally, see James W. Ceaser, *Nature and History in American Political Development* (Cambridge, MA: Harvard University Press, 2006), 20–59.

10. See, for instance, James Q. Wilson, *Political Organizations* (New York: Basic Books, 1973).

11. Theodore R. Marmor, *The Politics of Medicare*, 2nd ed. (Hawthorne, NY: Aldine de Gruyter, 2000), 3–21.

12. Wilson, *Political Organizations*, 332.

13. Ibid. See also: Daniel P. Moynihan, *The Politics of a Guaranteed Income* (New York: Random House, 1973).

14. U.S. Congress, House Committee on Ways and Means, "Medical Care for the Aged," executive hearings, 89th Cong., 1st Sess., January 28, 1965 (Washington, DC: U.S. Government Printing Office, 1965), 123–124.

15. Jonathan Oberlander, *The Political Life of Medicare* (Chicago: University of Chicago Press, 2003), 47–48.

16. Medicare has only had two enduring expansions. New coverage for end-stage renal disease and the disabled was added in 1972 and prescription drugs followed in 2003.

17. The definitive account of the MCCA is Richard Himelfarb, *Catastrophic Politics: The Rise and Fall of the Medicare Catastrophic Coverage Act of 1988* (University Park: Pennsylvania State University Press, 1995). See also Julie Rovner, "Congress's 'Catastrophic' Attempt to Fix Medicare," in *Intensive Care: How Congress Shapes Health Policy*, edited by Thomas E. Mann and Norman Ornstein (Washington, DC: American Enterprise Institute and Brookings Institution, 1995), 145-178; Thomas Rice, Katherine Desmond, and Jon Gabel, "The Medicare Catastrophic Coverage Act: A Post-mortem," *Health Affairs* 9.3 (1990): 75-87; "Reforming the American Welfare State: ERISA and the Medicare Catastrophic Coverage Act," in Eric M. Patashnik, *Reforms at Risk: What Happens after Major Policy Changes Are Enacted* (Princeton, NJ: Princeton University Press, 2008), 72-90; Oberlander, *The Political Life of Medicare*, 65-73.

18. Ronald Reagan, "Statement on the Proposed Catastrophic Health Insurance Legislation," February 12, 1987, http://www.presidency.ucsb.edu/ws/?pid=33679; Rovner, "Congress's 'Catastrophic' Attempt to Fix Medicare," 163.

19. U.S. Congress, House Committee on Ways and Means, Subcommittee on Health, "Catastrophic Illness Expenses" (Washington, DC: U.S. Government Printing Office, 1987), 141.

20. Rovner, "Congress's 'Catastrophic' Attempt to Fix Medicare," 158-159.

21. U.S. Congress, Senate, *Congressional Record*, 101st Cong, 1st Sess. (1989), S12871. See also Rice, Desmond, and Gabel, "The Medicare Catastrophic Coverage Act: A Post-mortem," 77.

22. Himelfarb, *Catastrophic Politics*, 40-44, and 80.

23. Jennifer O'Sullivan, "Medicare Catastrophic Coverage Act of 1988 (PL 100-360)," Congressional Research Service, Library of Congress, March 3, 1989, 20.

24. Himelfarb, *Catastrophic Politics*, 73.

25. Associated Press, "House Panel Leader Jeered by Elderly in Chicago," *New York Times*, August 19, 1989, A8.

26. Himelfarb, *Catastrophic Politics*, 62.

27. Rovner, "Congress's 'Catastrophic' Attempt to Fix Medicare," 172.

28. U.S. Bipartisan Commission on Comprehensive Health Care, *A Call for Action, Final Report* (Washington, DC: U.S. Government Printing Office, 1990); John D. Rockefeller, IV, "The Pepper Commission Report on Comprehensive Health Care," *New England Journal of Medicine* 323 (1990): 1005-1007.

29. U.S. Bipartisan Commission on Comprehensive Health Care, *A Call for Action*, 13-14.

30. Ibid., 14.

31. Ibid., 16.

32. Ibid., 17.

33. Mitchell Locin, "A Price Tag for National Health Plan," *Chicago Tribune*, September 25, 1990.

34. Joshua M. Wiener, Carroll L. Estes, Susan M. Goldenson, and Sheryl C. Goldberg, "What Happened to Long-Term Care in the Health Reform Debate of 1993-1994? Lessons for the Future," *The Milbank Quarterly* 79.2 (2001): 210.

35. Ibid.

36. Ibid.

37. Jacob S. Hacker, *The Road to Nowhere: The Genesis of President Clinton's Plan for Health Security* (Princeton, NJ: Princeton University Press, 1996); Theda Skocpol, *Health Care Reform and the Turn against Government* (New York: W. W. Norton, 1997).

38. Paul Pierson, "Policy Feedbacks" and Political Change: Contrasting Reagan and Thatcher's Pension-Reform Initiatives," *Studies in American Political Development* 6 (1992): 359-390; Theda Skocpol, *Protecting Soldiers and Mothers: The Political Origins of Social Policy in the United States* (Cambridge, MA: Harvard University Press, 1992).

39. Thomas A. Birkland, *Lessons of Disaster: Policy Change after Catastrophic Events* (Washington, DC: Georgetown University Press, 2006); Peter J. May, "Policy Learning and Failure," *Journal of Public Policy* 12.4 (1992): 331-354.

40. Weiner, Estes, Goldenson, and Goldberg, "What Happened to Long-Term Care in the Health Reform Debate of 1993-1994? Lessons for the Future," 241.

41. Ibid.

42. Interview with aging advocate, February 24, 2012.

43. Ibid.

44. David Blumenthal and James A. Morone, *The Heart of Power: Health and Politics in the Oval Office* (Berkeley: University of California Press, 2010), 8, 413.

45. Interview with former Department of Health and Human Services official, November 16, 2012.

46. Interview with aging advocate, February 24, 2012.

47. Kimberly J. Morgan and Andrea Louise Campbell, *The Delegated Welfare State: Medicare, Markets, and the Governance of Social Policy* (New York: Oxford University Press, 2011); Thomas R. Oliver, Philip R. Lee, and Helene L. Lipton, "A Political History of Medicare and Prescription Drug Coverage," *The Milbank Quarterly* 82.2 (2004): 283-354. This lesson has been reinforced yet again by the fallout over the Affordable Care Act's individual mandate. Though the provision passed muster with the Supreme Court, as of this writing, it remains unpopular with the American public.

48. Interview with aging advocate, February 24, 2012.

49. Weiner, Estes, Goldenson, and Goldberg, "What Happened to Long-Term Care in the Health Reform Debate of 1993-1994? Lessons for the Future," 235, 241-243.

CHAPTER 4

1. Theodore Lowi, *The End of Liberalism* (New York: W. W. Norton, 1979); Hugh Heclo, "Issue Networks and the Executive Establishment," in *The New American Political System*, edited by Anthony King (Washington, DC: American Enterprise Institute, 1978), 87-124; Frank R. Baumgartner and Beth Leech, *Basic Interests: The*

Importance of Groups in Politics and in Political Science (Princeton, NJ: Princeton University Press, 1998).

2. Christine Day, *What Older Americans Think: Interest Groups and Aging Policy* (Princeton, NJ: Princeton University Press, 1990); Ken Kollman, *Outside Lobbying: Public Opinion and Interest Group Strategies* (Princeton, NJ: Princeton University Press, 1998); Charles R. Morris, *The AARP: America's Most Powerful Lobby and the Clash of Generations* (New York: Times Books, 1996).

3. Interview with aging advocate, February 22, 2012.

4. Ibid.

5. Interview with aging advocate, February 24, 2012.

6. Interview with aging advocate, February 22, 2012.

7. Susan Rogers and Harriet Komisar, "Who Needs Long-Term Care?" Georgetown University Long-Term Care Financing Project, 2003, http://hpi.georgetown.edu/ltc/papers.html.

8. For other accounts of the CLASS Act, see: Howard Gleckman, "The Rise and Fall of the CLASS Act: What Lessons Can We Learn?" in *Universal Coverage of Long-Term Care in the United States: Can We Get There From Here?*, edited by Douglas Wolf and Nancy Folbre (New York: Russell Sage Foundation, 2012), 37–60; Robert B. Hudson, "The CLASS Promise in the Context of American Long-Term Care Policy," in *Universal Coverage of Long-Term Care in the United States*, edited by Douglas Wolf and Nancy Folbre (New York: Russell Sage Foundation, 2012), 61–78; Barbara Manard, "Dueling Talking Points: Technical Issues in Constructing and Passing the CLASS Act," *Public Policy and Aging Report* 20.2 (2010): 21–27; Robert B. Hudson, ed., "Bringing CLASS to Long-Term Care through the Affordable Care Act," *Public Policy & Aging Report* 20.2 (2010).

9. For more on the public option for health insurance that was considered for the Affordable Care Act, see John E. McDonough, *Inside National Health Reform* (Berkeley: University of California Press, 2011), 134–137.

10. Edward Kennedy, Tom Harkin, John Dingell, and Frank Pallone, "Kennedy, Harkin, Dingell, Pallone Introduce CLASS ACT: New Bipartisan Insurance Program Would Help Those with Severe Functional Impairments Gain Independence," Press Release, July 10, 2007.

11. Recipients would have had broad discretion in using the cash benefit. They could, for instance, have made home improvements like building wheelchair ramps or handicap-accessible showers. They might also have used the money to hire a health aide or family member to provide care at home. And while CLASS was not primarily focused on financing nursing home stays, the benefit could have also been used to defray institutional costs. Kennedy, et al., "Kennedy, Harkin, Dingell, Pallone Introduce CLASS ACT"; Joanne Kenen, "Health Policy Brief: The CLASS Act," *Health Affairs*, May 12, 2011, http://healthaffairs.org/healthpolicybriefs/brief_pdfs/healthpolicybrief_46.pdf; Patient Protection and Affordable Care Act, Public Law 111–148 (2010).

12. "CLASS Act," S.1951, 109th Cong. (2005). Charles Grassley (R-IA) had been Kennedy's initial Republican partner, but he withdrew to work on tax credits for the purchase of private insurance. Kaiser Family Foundation, "The Sleeper in

Health Reform: Long-Term Care and the CLASS Act," October 20, 2009, http://kaiserfamilyfoundation.files.wordpress.com/2013/01/102009_kff_class_act_transcript_final.pdf.

13. "CLASS Act," S.1758, 110th Cong. (2007); "Community Living Assistance Services and Supports Act," H.R.3001, 110th Cong. (2007). Having lost reelection, DeWine was no longer in the Senate. In 2009, Kennedy and Pallone reintroduced CLASS as stand-alone legislation, though inserting it into health reform was the central objective. "Community Living Assistance Services and Supports Act," S.697, 111th Cong. (2009); "Community Living Assistance Services and Supports Act," H.R.1721, 111th Cong. (2009).

14. U.S. Congress, Senate, *Congressional Record*, 110th Cong., 1st Sess. (July 10, 2007), S8948–S8949.

15. U.S. Congress, Senate, *Congressional Record*, 111th Cong., 1st Sess. (December 4, 2009), S12360.

CHAPTER 5

1. Interview with Democratic congressional staffer, February 21, 2012.

2. Interview with Democratic congressional staffers, February 24, 2012; phone interview with Democratic congressional staffer, March 9, 2012.

3. Interview with Democratic congressional staffers, February 24, 2012.

4. Phone interview with Democratic congressional staffer, March 9, 2012.

5. Interview with Democratic congressional staffers, February 24, 2012.

6. Phone interview with Democratic congressional staffer, March 9, 2012.

7. Ibid.

8. Interview with Democratic congressional staffers, February 24, 2012.

9. "Repeal the CLASS Entitlement Act," S.720, 112th Cong. (2011); U.S. Congress, Senate Committee on Health, Education, Labor and Pensions, "Community Services and Supports: Planning Across the Generations," 110th Cong., 1st Sess. (2007), 47, http://www.help.senate.gov/hearings/hearing/?id=0d2d8b6b-bda4-f2eb-74e7-6357d7588365.

10. Interview with Republican congressional staffer, February 24, 2012.

11. Interview with Democratic congressional staffer, February 21, 2012.

12. Interview with Republican congressional staffer, February 24, 2012.

13. HELP's chair duties were actually divided among Dodd, Harkin, and other members, but Dodd carried the gavel for health-care legislation.

14. Richard S. Foster, email to Jennifer M. Snow, May 19, 2009, http://www.thune.senate.gov/public/_files/ClassAct/ExhibitA.pdf.

15. Douglas W. Elmendorf, letter to Kay R. Hagan, July 6, 2009, http://www.cbo.gov/ftpdocs/104xx/doc10436/07-06-CLASSAct.pdf. See also: Elmendorf, letter to Edward M. Kennedy, July 2, 2009, http://www.cbo.gov/sites/default/files/cbofiles/ftpdocs/104xx/doc10431/07-02-helpltr.pdf.

16. Elmendorf, letter to Hagan, July 6, 2009.

17. Jill Gotts, email to Susan N. Hill et al., June 29, 2009, http://www.thune.senate.gov/public/_files/ClassAct/ExhibitB.pdf.

18. Gotts, email to Hill et al., July 8, 2009, http://www.thune.senate.gov/public/_files/ClassAct/ExhibitB.pdf.

19. U.S. Congress, Senate Committee on Health, Education, Labor, and Pensions Committee, "Senate HELP Committee Health Care Bill Markup—Day 8," July 7, 2009, https://www.c-span.org/video/?287499-1/health-care-reform-legislation-markup-day-8.

20. Ibid.

21. Ibid.

22. Interview with aging advocate, February 22, 2012.

23. Interview with aging advocate, February 24, 2012; interview with Democratic congressional staffer, February 29, 2012. See also: John E. McDonough, *Inside National Health Reform* (Berkeley: University of California Press, 2011), 244–245.

24. Interview with aging advocate, February 24, 2012.

25. Interview with Democratic congressional staffer, February 21, 2012; interview with Republican congressional staffer, February 23, 2012; interview with Republican congressional staffer, February 24, 2012; phone interview with Republican congressional staffer, March 1, 2012.

26. Sarah Kliff, "Meet the Senator Who Killed the CLASS Act," *Washington Post: Wonkblog*, October 18, 2011, http://www.washingtonpost.com/blogs/ezra-klein/post/meet-the-senator-who-killed-the-class-act/2011/10/18/gIQAhe7huL_blog.html.

27. Oliver Wyman, "Actuarial Analysis of the Community Living Assistance Services and Supports Act," AARP Report, March 3, 2008, http://www.thune.senate.gov/public/_files/ClassAct/ExhibitC.pdf.

28. Kaiser Family Foundation, "The Sleeper in Health Reform: Long-Term Care and the CLASS Act," October 20, 2009, http://kaiserfamilyfoundation.files.wordpress.com/2013/01/102009_kff_class_act_transcript_final.pdf.

29. Foster, email to Gotts, July 9, 2009; Gotts, email to Amy Hall, August 24, 2009, http://www.thune.senate.gov/public/_files/ClassAct/ExhibitB.pdf. Just over a month after sending his July 9 email, Foster sent two follow-up emails to ensure that his concerns had been communicated to Garner and the rest of the HELP staff. Foster, email to Gotts, August 14, 2009, http://www.thune.senate.gov/public/_files/ClassAct/ExhibitF.pdf.

30. The CBO estimated 3.5 percent of eligible individuals would enroll in CLASS. CMS estimated 2 percent. Garner used the more optimistic 5 percent figure. Elmendorf, letter to Thomas Harkin, November 25, 2009, http://www.cbo.gov/sites/default/files/cbofiles/ftpdocs/108xx/doc10823/class_additional_information_harkin_letter.pdf; Foster, "Estimated Financial Effects of the 'Patient Protection and Affordable Care Act,' as Passed by the Senate on December 24, 2009," https://www.cms.gov/Research-Statistics-Data-and-Systems/Research/ActuarialStudies/downloads/S_PPACA_2010-01-08.pdf; Kaiser Family Foundation, "The Sleeper in Health Reform: Long-Term Care and the CLASS Act."

31. Foster, email to Gotts, July 9, 2009.

32. Kaiser Family Foundation, "The Sleeper in Health Reform," 30–33.

33. Ibid., 30–31.

34. Ibid., 31, 32.

35. Ibid., 81.

36. Ibid., 31.

37. Numerous and repeated inquires about and attempts to acquire this study, learn more about how it was conducted, and identify the lead investigator proved unsuccessful.

38. P. J. Eric Stallard and Steven Schoonveld, "Actuarial Issues and Policy Implications of a Federal Long-Term Care Insurance Program," http://www.actuary.org/pdf/health/class_july09.pdf.

39. Elmendorf, letter to Harkin.

40. A study of CLASS released nearly a year after the Affordable Care Act became law came to broadly similar conclusions, including a finding that an average premium would run $194. Alicia H. Munnell and Josh Hurwitz, "What Is 'CLASS'? And Will It Work?" Center for Retirement Research at Boston College, 11-3 (February 2011), http://crr.bc.edu/wp-content/uploads/2011/02/IB_11-3-508.pdf.

41. Repeal CLASS Working Group, "CLASS' Untold Story: Taxpayers, Employers, and States on the Hook for Flawed Entitlement Program," 2011, http://www.thune.senate.gov/public/_cache/files/f03d8200-bfa4-4891-8a4c-aa78a54e2de0/C36C5CAFE5E1079F63B5508E247BC5C1.class-untold-story.pdf.

CHAPTER 6

1. This general concept is explored in a variety of settings in Richard H. Thaler and Cass R. Sunstein, *Nudge: Improving Decisions about Health, Wealth, and Happiness* (New Haven, CT: Yale University Press, 2008).

2. Interview with Democratic congressional staffer, April 23, 2014.

3. Kent Conrad, Joe Lieberman, Mary Landrieu, Evan Bayh, Blanche Lincoln, Ben Nelson, and Mark Warner, letter to Harry Reid, October 23, 2009, http://www.politico.com/pdf/PPM145_senate_class_act_letter.pdf.

4. Conrad et al., letter to Reid.

5. CBS News/AP, "Long-Term Care Program Gains Momentum," *CBS News*, October 27, 2009, http://www.cbsnews.com/news/long-term-care-program-gains-momentum/.

6. Lori Montgomery, "Proposed Long-Term Insurance Program Raises Questions," *Washington Post*, October 27, 2009, http://articles.washingtonpost.com/2009-10-27/politics/36874585_1_larry-minnix-long-term-care-insurance-program.

7. Shawn Tully, "The Crazy Math of Health-Care Reform," CNNMoney.com, September 3, 2009, http://money.cnn.com/2009/09/03/news/economy/health_care_class_act.fortune/index.htm.

8. Steven Brill, *America's Bitter Pill: Money, Politics, Backroom Deals, and the Fight to Fix Our Broken Healthcare System* (New York: Random House, 2015), 170.

9. Barack Obama, "Remarks by the President after Meeting with Senate Democrats," White House Office of the Press Secretary, December 15, 2009, http://www.whitehouse.gov/the-press-office/remarks-president-after-meeting-with-senate-democrats.

10. Montgomery, "Proposed Long-Term Insurance Program Raises Questions."

11. U.S. Department of Health and Human Services, "CLASS: Suggested Technical Corrections," 2010, http://www.thune.senate.gov/public/_files/ClassAct/ExhibitQ.pdf; U.S. Department of Health and Human Services, "A Report on the Actuarial, Marketing, and Legal Analyses of the CLASS Program," 2011, http://aspe.hhs.gov/daltcp/reports/2011/class/index.shtml.

12. Interview with Obama administration official, February 28, 2012.

13. Interview with Democratic congressional staffer, February 21, 2012.

14. Douglas W. Elmendorf, letter to Harry Reid, November 18, 2009, http://www.cbo.gov/sites/default/files/cbofiles/ftpdocs/107xx/doc10731/reid_letter_11_18_09.pdf.

15. Phone interview with Democratic congressional staffer, February 29, 2012.

16. U.S. Congress, Senate, *Congressional Record*, 111th Cong, 1st Sess. (December 4, 2009), S12394.

17. Ibid., S12389, S12394-5.

18. Ibid., S12389-90.

19. Ibid., S12375.

20. Ibid., S12360.

21. Ibid., S12382.

22. Interview with Democratic congressional staffer, February 21, 2012.

23. When a piece of legislation is brought to the Senate floor, unanimous consent agreements are commonly used to bypass normal chamber rules. They are negotiated on a bill-by-bill basis and establish the rules for a given piece of legislation—issues such as the amount of time for debate, allowable types of amendments, and the threshold for passing amendments.

24. Phone interview with Democratic congressional staffer, February 29, 2012.

25. A conference committee is the standard process in which discrepancies between the House and Senate versions of a bill are ironed out. A single piece of legislation is produced, and each chamber then holds one final vote on identical bills. The conference committee for health reform differed from the norm in that it consisted exclusively of Democrats. This partisan approach was chosen by Senate Majority Leader Reid because he had sufficient votes to pass health reform without any Republican support and wanted to avoid GOP attempts to delay the process.

26. The final Senate vote was 60-39. That tally included two independents—Lieberman and Bernie Sanders (VT)—who caucused with the Democrats. Republican Jim Bunning (KY) did not cast a vote.

27. The Major Party Index, for instance, routinely places Massachusetts among the most Democratic states. See: James W. Ceaser and Robert P. Saldin, "A New Measure of Party Strength," *Political Research Quarterly* 58.2 (2005): 245-256.

28. Sally Jacobs, "Modeling Years Gave Scott Brown a Boost," *Boston Globe*, October 24, 2012, http://www.boston.com/news/politics/2012/2012/10/23/scott-brown-modeling-years/jumcPmY74StGiXtubQPEcJ/story.html.

29. Tracey D. Samuelson, "Coakley Concedes Race: Five Lessons from Her Campaign," *Christian Science Monitor*, January 20, 2010, http://www.csmonitor.com/USA/Politics/2010/0120/Coakley-concedes-race-five-lessons-from-her-campaign; Boris Shor, "Scott Brown Is a More Liberal Republican than Dede Scozzafava,"

http://research.bshor.com/2010/01/15/scott-brown-is-a-more-liberal-republican-than-dede-scozzafava/; "Massachusetts Senate – Special Election," *Real Clear Politics*, http://www.realclearpolitics.com/epolls/2010/senate/ma/massachusetts_senate_special_election-1144.html.

30. "Massachusetts Senate – Special Election," *Real Clear Politics*.

31. "Nightside with Dan Rea," January 15, 2010, https://www.youtube.com/watch?v=OmNpcMHwOa8.

32. Paul Kane and Karl Vick, "Republican Wins Kennedy's Seat," *Washington Post*, January 20, 2010, http://articles.washingtonpost.com/2010-01-20/politics/36855989_1_senate-seat-republican-scott-brown-obama-aides.

33. Stephanie Condon, "Scott Brown Win Shakes Up Health Care Fight," *CBS New*, January 20, 2010, http://www.cbsnews.com/8301-503544_162-6119035-503544/scott-brown-win-shakes-up-health-care-fight/.

34. Glen Johnson and Liz Sidoti, "Massachusetts Senate Race Results: Scott Brown Defeats Martha Coakley," *Huffington Post*, January 19, 2010, http://www.huffingtonpost.com/2010/01/19/massachusetts-senate-race_1_n_429033.html.

35. Technically, the parliamentarian only offers advice, and it could, at least in theory, be rejected. But as a matter of practice, if the parliamentarian says a provision should be excluded, it is.

36. Sheryl Gay Stolberg, "Parliamentarian in Role as Health Bill Referee," *New York Times*, March 13, 2010, http://www.nytimes.com/2010/03/14/us/politics/14rules.html?_r=0; *New York Times*, "Refereeing the Health Care Debate," March 5, 2010, http://www.nytimes.com/2010/03/06/opinion/06sat4.html?ref=alansfrumin.

37. Stolberg, "Parliamentarian in Role as Health Bill Referee."

38. John Stanton, "Police Concerned about Parliamentarian's Safety," *Roll Call*, March 25, 2010, http://www.rollcall.com/news/-44688-1.html.

39. CLASS was officially repealed a little over a year later as part of the American Taxpayer Relief Act of 2012, also known as the "fiscal cliff" bill. Kathleen Sebelius, "The CLASS Program," *Huffington Post*, October 14, 2011, http://www.huffingtonpost.com/sec-kathleen-sebelius/the-class-program_b_1011270.html.

40. Major Garrett, "CLASS Act? The Obama Administration Has Put a Stake in the Heart of an Important Health Provision: What It Says about the White House and Washington," *National Journal*, October 20, 2011.

41. Garrett, "CLASS Act?"

CHAPTER 7

1. George W. Bush, "Remarks on Signing the Economic Growth and Tax Relief Reconciliation Act of 2001," June 7, 2001, http://www.presidency.ucsb.edu/ws/index.php?pid=45820&st=&st1=.

2. Jacob S. Hacker and Paul Pierson, "Abandoning the Middle: The Bush Tax Cuts and the Limits of Democratic Control," *Perspectives on Politics* 3.1 (2005): 33; Citizens for Tax Justice, "Year-by-Year Analysis of the Bush Tax Cuts Shows Growing Tilt to the Very Rich," June 12, 2002, http://www.ctj.org/html/gwb0602.htm.

3. Bush, "2001 Address to Congress," *Washington Post*, February 27, 2001, http://www.washingtonpost.com/wp-srv/onpolitics/transcripts/bushtext022701.htm.

See also, for example, Bush, "Remarks in Sioux Falls, South Dakota," March 9, 2001, http://www.presidency.ucsb.edu/ws/?pid=45764; Bush, "Remarks on Signing the Economic Growth and Tax Relief Reconciliation Act of 2001."

4. Hacker and Pierson, "Abandoning the Middle," 43.

5. Mona Lewandoski, "The Bush Tax Cuts of 2001 and 2003: A Brief Legislative History," Harvard Law School Federal Budget Policy Seminar, May 6, 2008, 22, http://www.law.harvard.edu/faculty/hjackson/2001-2003TaxCuts_37.pdf; Joel Friedman, Richard Kogan, and Robert Greenstein, "New Tax-Cut Law Ultimately Costs as Much as Bush Plan," Center on Budget and Policy Priorities, June 27, 2001, http://www.cbpp.org/archives/5-26-01tax.htm.

6. Richard Kogan and Joel Friedman, "New Tax Cut Law Uses Gimmicks to Mask Costs; Ultimate Price Tag Likely to be $800 Billion to $1 Trillion," Center on Budget and Policy Priorities, June 1, 2003, http://www.cbpp.org/archives/5-22-03tax.htm.

7. William G. Gale and Peter R. Orszag, "Sunsets in the Tax Code," *Tax Notes*, June 9, 2003, 1557.

8. Ibid., 1557–1558.

9. Friedman, Kogan, and Greenstein, "New Tax-Cut Law Ultimately Costs as Much as Bush Plan."

10. Hacker and Pierson, "Abandoning the Middle," 45–46.

11. Ibid., 35 and 46.

12. Bush, "State of the Union Address," January 28, 2003. See, in general: Jonathan Oberlander, "Through the Looking Glass: The Politics of the Medicare Prescription Drug, Improvement, and Modernization Act," *Journal of Health Politics, Policy, and Law* 32.2 (Apr. 2007): 187–219; Thomas R. Oliver, Philip R. Lee, and Helene L. Lipton, "A Political History of Medicare and Prescription Drug Coverage," *The Milbank Quarterly* 82.2 (2004): 283–354.

13. Congressional Budget Office, *A Detailed Description of CBO's Cost Estimate for the Medicare Prescription Drug Benefit* (July 2004).

14. Congressional Budget Office, "Cost Estimate for H.R. 1, the Medicare Prescription Drug, Improvement, and Modernization Act of 2003," November 20, 2003. See also: Donald B. Marron, "Understanding CBO Health Cost Estimates," *Backgrounder*, No. 2298, July 15,2009.

15. Amy Goldstein, "Higher Medicare Costs Suspected for Months," *Washington Post*, January 31, 2004, A1.

16. Richard S. Foster, "The Hot Seat," *Contingencies*, November–December 2004, 26, http://www.contingencies.org/novdec04/coverstory.pdf.

CHAPTER 8

1. Aaron Wildavsky, *Speaking Truth to Power* (Boston: Little, Brown 1979). See, especially, chapter 2: "Strategic Retreat on Objectives: Learning from Failure in American Public Policy."

2. James Madison, "Federalist 51," *The Federalist Papers*, 1788; Madison "Federalist 62," *The Federalist Papers*, 1788.

3. See, for instance: Gregory Koger, *Filibustering: A Political History of Obstruction in the House and Senate* (Chicago: University of Chicago Press, 2010).

4. Dan L. Crippen, letter to John M. Spratt Jr., *Congressional Record – House*, Vol. 145 (1999), Part 16, 23010–23016.

5. Truth in Budgeting and Social Security Protection Act of 2005, S.568, 109th Cong. (2005). Very similar legislation was also introduced in the 107th and 108th Congresses.

6. Eric M. Patashnik, "Ideas, Inheritances, and the Dynamics of Budgetary Change," *Governance: An International Journal of Policy and Administration* 12.2 (1999): 147; Paul Pierson, "The Deficit and the Politics of Domestic Reform," in *The Social Divide: Political Parties and the Future of Activist Government*, edited by Margaret Weir (Washington, DC: Brookings Institution Press, 1999), 127. See also: Eric M. Patashnik, "Congress and the Budget since 1974," in *The American Congress: The Building of Democracy*, edited by Julian E. Zelizer (New York: Houghton Mifflin, 2004), 668–686.

7. "Retirement Age: Background," Social Security, http://www.ssa.gov/retirement/background.htm; Gayle L. Reznik, Dave Shoffner, and David A. Weaver, "Coping with the Demographic Challenge: Fewer Children and Living Longer," *Social Security Bulletin* 66.4 (2005–2006), http://www.ssa.gov/policy/docs/ssb/v66n4/v66n4p37.html.

8. For a critique of the assumptions and methodology employed by the CBO and Foster, see: Barbara Manard, "Dueling Talking Points: Technical Issues in Constructing and Passing the CLASS Act," *Public Policy and Aging Report* 20.2 (2010): 21–27.

9. Interview with aging advocate, February 24, 2012.

10. Manard, "Dueling Talking Points," 26.

11. Alicia H. Munnell and Josh Hurwitz, "What Is 'CLASS'? And Will It Work?" Center for Retirement Research at Boston College, February 2011, Number 11-3, http://crr.bc.edu/wp-content/uploads/2011/02/IB_11-3-508.pdf.

12. Munnell and Hurwitz, "What Is 'CLASS'? And Will It Work," 5; Douglas W. Elmendorf, letter to Thomas Harkin, November 25, 2009, http://www.cbo.gov/sites/default/files/cbofiles/ftpdocs/108xx/doc10823/class_additional_information_harkin_letter.pdf; Richard S. Foster, "Estimated Financial Effects of the 'Patient Protection and Affordable Care Act,' as Passed by the Senate on December 24, 2009," https://www.cms.gov/Research-Statistics-Data-and-Systems/Research/ActuarialStudies/downloads/S_PPACA_2010-01-08.pdf; Kaiser Family Foundation, "The Sleeper in Health Reform: Long-Term Care and the CLASS Act," October 20, 2009, http://kaiserfamilyfoundation.files.wordpress.com/2013/01/102009_kff_class_act_transcript_final.pdf.

13. Munnell and Hurwitz, "What Is 'CLASS'? And Will It Work," 4–5. They also ran an implausible but illustrative model in which there was an individual mandate to participate in CLASS and found that the average monthly premium would be $94. And while that's way below private market offerings, it's way above the premium levels that the optional CLASS program had long been predicated on. Moreover, a $94 monthly premium would not be seen as affordable for many Americans.

14. Sandra R. Levitsky, *Caring for Our Own: Why There Is No Political Demand for New American Social Welfare Rights* (New York: Oxford University Press, 2014).

15. Eric M. Patashnik, *Reforms at Risk: What Happens after Major Policy Changes Are Enacted* (Princeton, NJ: Princeton University Press, 2008), 19, 155. Italics in original.

16. Howard Gleckman, "Long-Term Care Financing Reform: Lessons from the U.S. and Abroad," February 2010; Andrea Louise Campbell and Kimberly J. Morgan, "Federalism and the Politics of Old-Age Care in Germany and the United States," *Comparative Political Studies* 38.8 (October 2005): 887–914.

17. Michael Cooper, "Conservatives Sowed Idea of Health Care Mandate, Only to Spurn It Later," *New York Times*, February 14, 2012, http://www.nytimes.com/2012/02/15/health/policy/health-care-mandate-was-first-backed-by-conservatives.html?_r=0.

18. See, for instance, James Q. Wilson, *Political Organizations* (New York: Basic Books, 1973), 332.

19. David Stevenson, Richard G. Frank, and Jocelyn Tau, "Private Long-Term Care Insurance and State Tax Incentives," *Inquiry* 46.3 (2009): 305–321; Gleckman, "Long-Term Care Financing Reform: Lessons from the U.S. and Abroad," 19.

20. Stephen A. Moses, "The Long-Term Health Care Crisis: How Can We Solve It?" April 27, 2000, http://www.heritage.org/research/lecture/how-to-deal-with-the-coming-crisis.

21. Senate Committee on Health, Education, Labor and Pensions, "Community Services and Supports: Planning Across the Generations," 110th Congress, July 10, 2007.